I0712081

INTERMITTENT

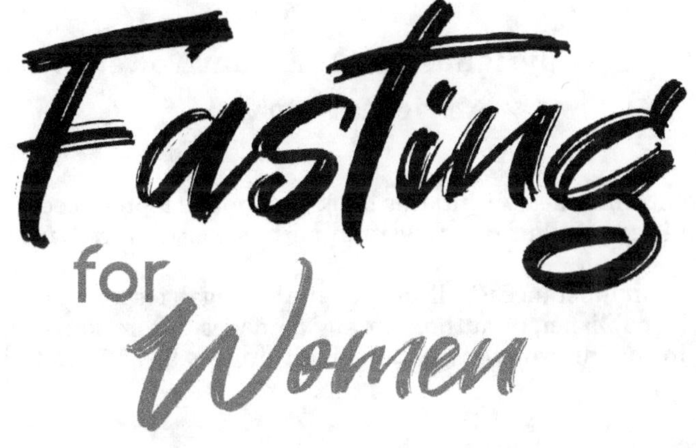

Fasting
for
Women

Learn to Improve your Health.
Step by Step Guide for Beginners, Start Your
New Lifestyle & Weight Loss, for Women & Over 50.
Useful and Instant Recipes.

MELANY POWER

Title:
Intermittent Fasting for Women

MELANY POWER

Table of Contents

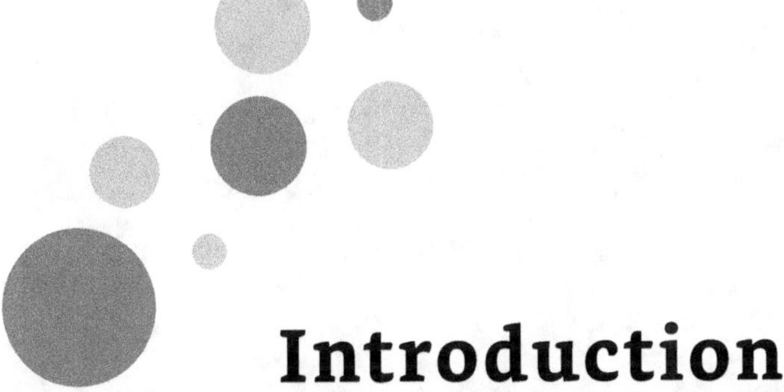

Introduction

Obesity and weight issues have become one of the biggest concerns these days. Obesity-related deaths form the major portion of preventable deaths in the US. Obesity is a big problem for all groups and sections of society; however, it becomes an even bigger problem when it comes to women. For a woman, being fat means battling much more. It has severe psychological and social consequences other than physiological ones.

The society has never been fair to anyone. Since the very beginning of time, cherry picking the best has been the norm for every species and humans haven't been any different. Outcasting people on the basis of their looks, color, race, and physical structure has always been common. We have come a long way from the crude ways of the past, yet things haven't changed completely.

An obese person, in general, would find it very hard to leave a positive first impression. An obese or overweight woman would struggle even much harder.

We may like it or not but the world doesn't have a very kind view of the obese people. Most people think of obese people as lazy, stupid, ugly, and unhappy. They have to struggle to gain popularity in any real sense and easily get the stamp of being greedy and gross. Obesity brings depression along with it and the victims may feel unmotivated and unhealthy. However, for all that matters to other people, they think obesity is self-inflicted torture that obese people choose to bear. Most experts believe that weight bias in society is as prevalent as racism. In fact, a Yale University study found that obesity discrimination has increased by 66% in the past few years.

The bias against obese people is also very high even in the minds of healthcare professionals like doctors, nurses, and other medical professionals. They mostly believe that the reason for persistent weight gain is carelessness, indiscipline, lack of motivation and hard work in obese people. They are fat because they are not putting serious effort into losing weight. This is very far from the truth, as people with weight issues want it more than anyone else.

For women, the consequences of unwanted excess weight or obesity are far deeper. It burdens them with shame and rejection. Only a few may choose to accept the fact openly, but they do have an inferior image of themselves. Obese women generally battle with issues like low self-esteem, depression, and loneliness. Discrimination and prejudice against obese women are also exceptionally high even in their own circle.

This is one of the biggest reasons that obese women are obsessed with weight management. Men usually fail to understand these complexities or conveniently choose to ignore them. For a woman, an increase in weight is not just a difficulty of fitting in the old clothes, but it also means facing the stare of her friends. Not finding the same level of acceptance even among your own kind is the biggest humiliation one can face and it happens more often than people choose to accept.

The insane pace with which the weight loss industry has grown in the past few decades is a live testimony of the fact that obese people do recognize it as a problem. It isn't their ignorance of the problem but the futility of the solutions that have been a problem.

Therefore, we all, especially women, conclusively know that obesity or any kind of uncontrolled increase in weight is a problem. The percentage of men suffering from weight issues is higher than women, yet the memberships in weight control programs are dominated by women. Around 90% of weight watcher members are women. Women are more likely to start dieting, calorie restriction and exercise when they feel that they are gaining weight. Men generally tend to have a very laidback attitude on the same BMI. Women take an increase in weight very seriously.

They have been adopting even harsh methods to control weight. The methods have been harsh to the extent of punishment. Living without the favorite foods for months at length is a punishment. Coping on hundreds of calories short of daily need isn't an easy task. Eating only a specific type of food in order to avoid excess intake of calories is not a mean feat that anyone can pull off. Yet, women do it all the time. They have been doing it for years now. Sadly, they haven't worked well. The numbers say that obesity among women is increasing rapidly. In the US alone, more than 70% of the adult population is facing obesity and women are leading in this percentage.

Most of the weight loss methods like diets, pills, exercise, calorie restriction, etc. are difficult measures and give inconsistent results. Women start with great resolve but find themselves at sea when these methods stop showing results and become ineffective. It isn't the lack of commitment towards weight loss but lackluster performance of these measures.

Women are the biggest subscribers of all kinds of weight loss programs. They are more conscious even towards a slight increase in their weight. Yet, they experience slow fat loss as compared to men. They also face more physiological problems and hormonal changes due to weight gain. They are ready to put in all the time and effort in controlling the weight.

However, conventional weight loss measures have not been working and even if they show results, in the beginning, they seem to lose effect after a while. The kind of control and commitment required in most of the weight loss programs is harsh to the extent of punishment. Yet, women are ready to bear them as they know that an increase in weight can have even more significant effect. The actual problem lies in the way these measures treat weight gain.

Weight gain in any individual is simply not a result of an increase in the intake of calories. Although calories do play a major role in weight gain, they are not the only cause. One-solution-fits-all wouldn't work in this case. These measures are simply trying to control the symptoms while they completely ignore the root cause of the problem.

To have any effective restraint over excess weight and other metabolic issues in women, they need a way that will help in solving the problem from within. To be sustainable in the long run, it should be easy and practical.

CHAPTER

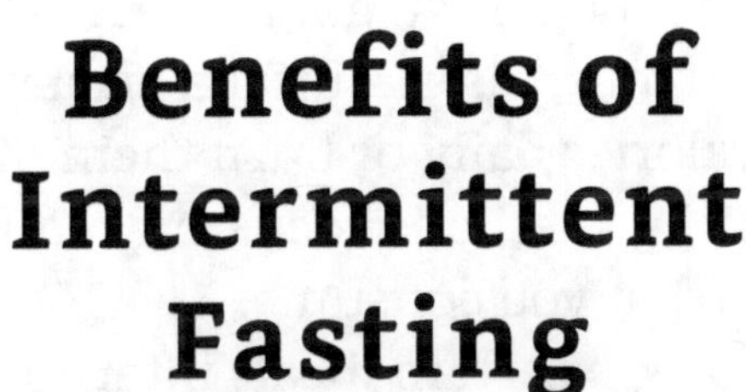

Benefits of Intermittent Fasting

Intermittent fasting is making headlines, because of the range of benefits that it provides. In this section, we will examine these benefits in greater detail.

Intermittent Fasting leads to Weight Loss

For any diet or weight loss method to work, you must monitor your calorie intake either you must consume fewer calories daily or burn them off regularly. Thus, all the fasting methods focus on reducing the number of calories that you consume.

If you skip certain meals intermittently, you consume fewer calories. For example, if you skip breakfast in the morning, you decrease your daily calorie intake by 500 calories. That is how intermittent fasting causes weight loss.

Intermittent fasting leads to the loss of body fat.

You might say that you want to lose weight. However, it is not the weight that you should focus on, but the extra body fat. This is important to mention because weight loss could also be triggered by a loss of muscle mass. However, that is not something you would want to achieve.

The idea is to get rid of excess body fat and not muscle mass. Losing muscle mass actually does not serve the purpose here. According to various studies, intermittent fasting helps you lose excess body fat rather than muscle mass. This is how it contributes to effective weight loss.

Intermittent fasting preserves muscle mass

Most of the weight loss routines available to us focus on losing both muscle mass and excess body fat. Losing muscle mass is undesirable because it could lead to dropping metabolic rates that could be harmful to your body.

Intermittent fasting can keep you from gaining weight during the holidays.

Weight gain is a steady process that occurs throughout the year. However, around the time of holidays like Christmas and Thanksgiving, and other vacation periods, the rate of weight gain increases dramatically!

This is the time when intermittent fasting could really help you. In fact, in these situations, alternate periods of eating and fasting could keep your calorie count in check and you do not have to worry about eating big for the other meals. So, even during your holidays, you could maintain a rather simple diet of intermittent fasting and you are good to go!

Intermittent fasting does not result in extreme hunger cravings

Unlike other fasting methods and techniques, intermittent fasting does not cause severe hunger cravings, which might cause you to overeat. Intermittent fasting controls your diet and hunger, so, you would be able to eat less without having major hunger cravings.

How does intermittent fasting control your hanger? IF keeps your hunger hormones at bay. Thus, they do not affect your body adversely.

What Do Studies Say?

An average human being must lose about 1600 - 1800 calories per day to lose weight. By skipping breakfast as a part of intermittent fasting, 30% of that target is already achieved.

Studies suggest that IF causes weight loss of about 4

- 7% near the waist circumference across a period of 24 weeks. This results in the loss of belly fat.

Usually, other dieting methods and restrictions can get rid of 25% of muscle mass but this is harmful to the body and not recommended. In contrast, intermittent fasting can remove only about 10% of muscle mass.

According to studies, fasting regularly causes hunger hormones to run into overdrive. However, since intermittent fasting requires you to alternate periods of fasting and eating, you do not get hunger cravings.

1.1
Intermittent Fasting Reduces the Risk of Type 2 Diabetes

Each person is unique with a unique combination and type of body structure. Thus, different people react differently to diabetes issues and symptoms. In effect, there are several different ways of treating type2 diabetes.

However, intermittent fasting is known to be more effective than other methods when it comes to reducing the risks of type 2 diabetes. Alternate periods of fasting and eating, help reduce the imbalance of glucose in the body.

What Do Studies Suggest?

It has been noted that people who restrict their diets by consuming their food only during certain times of the day while fasting during the rest of the day (while fasting during the rest of the day), seem to maintain their glucose levels more successfully.

If you consume your calories for the day during only certain times of the day for a period of eight days your insulin sensitivity will increase significantly. This will be accompanied by an increased pancreatic response to changing insulin levels. The earlier that you finish your meals, the greater the likelihood that your body will be at reduced risk of developing several different diseases. Furthermore, you will benefit from a reduction in blood pressure, oxidative stress and even reduced hunger cravings.

It is not enough to consume all your meals as early as possible. It is important to ensure that to meal timings are synchronized with the body's natural biological clock

There are many underlying benefits and concepts associated with intermittent fasting and its impact on type 2 diabetes. Controlling the glucose levels within the body is more convenient in the morning than in the evening. Thus, intermittent fasting, carried out during the morning (across eight hours) allows you to control the sugar content in the body more easily.

Many studies have been conducted in the recent past that explain the effect of intermittent fasting on maintaining the glucose levels in the body. On such study included research on eight men with prediabetes.

In this particular study, the eight men were asked to eat their breakfast between 6:30 and 8:30 a.m. Thereafter, they were provided with a 6-hour time frame during which they would have to finish the rest of the meals. They were required to fast during the rest of the day and not were not allowed to eat anything while carrying out their normal activities. As a result, all of them managed to finish their dinner by 3 p.m.

There was a second group involved in the same study. This group maintained their diet across a 12-hour time frame. They managed to eat the same kind of foods, at regular intervals.

The researchers found that the first group of people, the ones who could finish the entire diet within the 6-hour period had better insulin sensitivity.

What's more, it was also found that the pancreas reacts better to rising levels of insulin in the body. As a combination of these two factors, the body becomes better equipped to deal with varying levels of glucose.

The benefits of intermittent fasting do not end there. It has been observed that this type of diet reduces blood pressure in men.

Intermittent fasting decreases the risk of developing type 2 diabetes and hypertension. These health benefits, coupled with weight loss, illustrate how intermittent fasting is great for your overall health.

Intermittent Fasting Enhances

Brain Health

Let us begin this discussion by finding out what studies have discovered.

A study was conducted on mice where one was given free access to food while the other was kept on a brief intermittent fasting diet. It was found that the latter learned better and retained a better memory than the former one.

Another study using animals showed that intermittent fasting helps reduce inflammation in the brain and helps to lower the risk of many neurological disorders, (including Alzheimer's, and Parkinson's) and the risk of strokes.

These studies used animals and mammals, but some of the results can be applied to human beings. Neuroscience research has supported the fact that IF helps your brain in many ways. Some of them have been listed below.

Making BDNF

Brain-derived neurotrophic factor (BDNF) is an essential protein present in the brain that is responsible for the growth of new neurons. It enhances the communication process within the brain, and acts as a natural antidepressant.

Not just that, BDNF also helps the neurons to stay healthy for a longer time. Dementia, Alzheimer's and other brain-related problems are linked directly to low levels of BDNF in the brain.

Intermittent fasting increases the production of these proteins. A 400 increase in BDNF levels has been observed in people following IF.

Anti-Aging Effects

A group of ten people with cognitive impairment (loss of ability to think, recollect and memorize) were chosen for research. They had started showing early signs of Alzheimer's. Some changes were made to their lifestyle, one of which was to fast for 12-14 hours every night. After 3-6 months, nine out of the ten subjects had improved their cognitive abilities.

This study demonstrates that IF keeps your brain younger. It protects against the loss of structure and functionofneurons.Theslow-downofneurodegeneration also slows down the aging of the brain. You stay smarter and mentally active for a longer time if you fast regularly.

Seizure Reduction

Carbohydrates are considered the main fuel for the brain. Reports suggest that the brain uses more carbs when you are fasting than when you are not fasting. This leads to a significant reduction in the number of epileptic seizures. Therefore, IF plays a crucial role in decreasing the risk for epilepsy and abnormal functioning of the brain.

Decreased Brain Damage

Studies have shown that fasting increases BDNF, anti-oxidant and anti-inflammatory compounds in the brain. It also decreases brain damage and most importantly, protects a person from dying from a stroke. This is a big advantage that comes by simply opting for scheduled eating time. Since intermittent fasting only tells you to eat in a particular window in a day, the benefits that come along are much greater. Anyone would wish to prevent brain damage for as long as possible.

Improved Brain Function

Think about how exercise affects your muscles. Even a little workout makes them more efficient and healthier. The same thing happens with your brain when you are fasting. The brain cells are put under mild stress, which causes them to slowly adapt to the environment they are being forced into. This makes them more energy efficient and active.

Your body recovers from intense exercise by burning the extra fat and cleansing the cells. The brain does recover from fasting by entering the building phase. This improves brain function and neuronal connections.

Higher HGH

Human growth hormone (HGH) provides the following benefits to the human body:

Powerful anti-aging properties

Longevity

Neurogenesis (making new nerve cells and tissues)

Neuroprotection

Cognition

Cell repair

The health of brain cells

When a hormone is this essential for your body, it is sensible to focus on generating it at high levels. Intermittent fasting naturally boosts the HGH levels in your body. Taking this hormone from outside artificial sources is not the best for your body and is not recommended for a lot of reasons.

More Energy

You would know that mitochondria are known as the powerhouse of the cells. Each cell contains thousands of mitochondria that give them the power to carry out the body's functions. They are work like the batteries in your phone. Higher battery storage makes your phone last longer and works more efficiently. A higher number of mitochondria in the brain cells means more brain-power.

Studies have shown that intermittent fasting boosts mitochondrial biogenesis, the creation of new mitochondria.

Fasting results in several positive neurochemical changes in the brain cells that improve the cognitive function. Restricting calorie intake reduces inflammation in the brain and increases the production and growth of neurons in the brain. This is a big factor behind increasing your learning power and memory capacity. Studies have also indicated that fasting increases the ability of nerve cells to repair DNA.

Intermittent fasting doesn't just lead to weight loss and a healthy heart; it enhances brain health and function.

Intermittent Fasting Takes

Care of Your Heart

Based on a report published by the WHO (World Health Organization), each year, 17.9 million people around the world die due to cardiovascular diseases. This is about one-third of all deaths that occur in a year in the world. This shows that heart diseases are a serious problem today. People over the age of 45 years are affected the most by them.

Modifiable factors such as smoking, obesity, lack of physical activity, metabolism disorders, hypertension, poor diet, and high cholesterol, are some of the major factors that lead to the development of serious heart diseases in individuals. We call them modifiable because certain changes in a person's lifestyle can reduce the related risk. These changes include making adjustments like smoking cessation, increasing physical activity and maintaining proper body weight.

Obese people are usually the target of heart-related problems. Studies have found that fighting obesity can be a solution to all of them and it can be achieved by reducing a person's calorie intake and burning their extra-fat. The easiest way to achieve this is through intermittent fasting methods, which mainly focus on consuming meals within a strictly defined period.

It has been confirmed that an IF diet enhances the health of a person's heart. A healthy heart means longevity and a healthy body. This is due to the impact that IF has on various factors that increase the risk of catching a cardiovascular disease. Some of the major impacts have been discussed below:

Lowers Blood Pressure

High level of blood pressure, also known as hypertension, is the main reason behind a stroke or chronic kidney disease. Research and experiments have shown that fasting can help to reduce blood pressure.

Regular intake of high-calorie food leads to increased weight, cholesterol, and blood pressure. Strict dieting methods help to reduce the number of calories a person consumes daily. Intermittent fasting gives the body a long time to use the extra calories to provide energy to the body.

When you alternate eating with fasting, your body's food cravings decrease. Your body burns its excess calories to boost your metabolism and give you energy.

Lower blood pressure levels prevent any sort of heart problems from developing.

Reduces Cholesterol

The risk of having a heart attack is high in individuals with elevated cholesterol levels. These people who regularly consume oily and fries items, for example.

The human body undergoes a lot of internal transformations while fasting. Its metabolic processes improve. Various studies show that the level of total cholesterol (TC) triglycerides and low-density cholesterol (LDL) decrease when a person is fasting. This, in turn, results in limiting the risk of developing coronary heart disease.

Controls Diabetes

Diabetes is caused when the blood sugar levels and insulin resistance in person's body are dangerously high. Intermittent fasting improves blood sugar control, which is useful for those who are at risk of developing diabetes.

When you follow the 'fast and feast' method, insulin resistance decreases, and it becomes easier for the insulin to transport glucose from the blood to the cells more efficiently. Keeping the blood sugar and insulin levels under control goes a long way in ensuring a healthy heart.

Reduces Inflammation

Low levels of inflammation are very helpful for better health. A study performed on 50 healthy adults showed that one month of intermittent fasting decreased their inflammatory markers by a considerable amount. Although acute inflammation is a normal immune process, too much of anything is always harmful. That is why chronic levels may lead to the development of heart diseases.

Decreases the Risk of Metabolic Syndrome

Metabolic syndrome happens when a combination of conditions (high blood pressure, high blood sugar, high cholesterol, excess body fat) come together as a cluster. This increases the risk of heart disease, stroke or type 2 diabetes.

The whole process of intermittent fasting is effective because it burns the extra fat and mass stored in the body. This, in turn, greatly helps in maintaining a healthy cardiovascular system. All these positive changes change the concentration of metabolic biomarkers in the body, thus reducing the risk of metabolic syndrome.

A Healthy Heart is Important

The mortality rate is different in males and females. Studies show that the death rate is higher in men between the age of 45 and 59, while in women it becomes dominant after the age of 60. This is due to the effect of menopause on woman's heart.

All the causes of an unhealthy heart are linked to each other. Excessive fat, high cholesterol, increased blood pressure and sugar levels trigger one other. If one number changes, it causes others to change as well. Though this is bad for your health, you can turn this dependency upside down to your advantage. When you are fasting, your body looks for energy sources to boost metabolic activities. This is when the stored fat of your body comes into play. It is broken down and the energy in it is used by the blood.

When this fat burns, it decreases all other factors leading to an unhealthy heart. Even during your non-fasting period, you should eat food that regulates digestion and contributes to better heart health. Choose a nutritional diet that helps to diminish the level of your body fat. Doing this will help you to losing weight and prevent you from becoming obese. In short, intermittent fasting is a good way to ensure that you have a healthy heart.

The Truth about Intermittent Fasting

It all the rage, support, trendiness, and glamour associated with Intermittent Fasting, it's uncomplicated to get up and seek the truth behind all of it. After all, when you are looking forward to giving up your comfort zone and dedicatedly devote yourself to such a strict eating regime, you need to be sure about the results or pay-outs. You need to be sure that it's worth pursuing and is not just another millennial fad.

So, here are some answers to your intriguing questions: Is it even safe?

Intermittent fasting isn't a new fad. It has been around for years. In the Hindu religion, certain festivals require devotees to refrain from eating for the entire day. Ramadan is an Islamic holy month during which people don't consume food from sunrise to sunset. In Christianity, fasting occurs during Lent. So, it's safe to say that people have been practicing intermittent fasting in the past, and it hasn't caused any major serious complications.

Your body has enough energy stored in the fat cells to get you through the day without food and water. This won't even cause any major hormone imbalances either, thanks to the magical adaptability of our body when under stress.

But to ensure complete safety, you should pick the IF type that's suited to your body. If you're overweight, an 8-hour fast is always better than a 24-hour fast or 5:2 IF. Additionally, it's important to refuel your body with essential proteins, vitamins, minerals and lots of water after you finish fasting. This will ensure your body returns to normal and starts functioning the way it's supposed to.

Will I get too weak?

The simple answer is no. As stated previously, your body has stored enough calories in the fatty cells to get you through the fasting hours. When you fast, your body enters a state known as gluconeogenesis. This is when the liver creates its own glucose to keep your body running. You may temporarily experience dizziness, or fatigue (which is completely normal). Many professional athletes and experienced dieters even perform physical activities and hit the gym while fasting. So, you shouldn't be worrying about weakness.

How does it affect my metabolism?

Many people believe that IF negatively affects their metabolism. But when you lose weight, the body adapts and causes your metabolism to slow down. This is because losing weight is accompanied by the loss of muscle and fat, which provide the required calories during the fasting hours.

Your body goes into fasting mode only after 8 hours of fasting, when it enters the gluconeogenesis state. At this point, there is no glucose left in the liver, and the fat reserves are used. It is only after 24 to 48 hours that your body goes into starvation mode and over time, the metabolic rate decreases. The body does this as a defense mechanism.

Some studies have indicated that in the long-term, calorie restriction reduces the metabolic rate, but any major or minor complications are almost non-existent. More quality research is required to determinate the long-term effects of IF on metabolic rate, but until now it's been on the safe side.

Will it help me to lose weight?

All the protocols of IF should be diligently followed and correctly timed in order to ensure weight loss.

For example, when using the 16:8 intermittent fasting method, you should only consume food during the 8 hour window and fast for the remaining 16 hours. As a rule, you also need to refrain from eating, processed junk food, which can increase your calories.

While it definitely is a safe option for weight loss when done correctly, its effectiveness is still under scrutiny. Some studies have pointed out that it is an excellent weight-loss method, while others have found no significant cor-relatable evidence of it being better than traditional weight loss methods, such as exercise.

Is there any medical evidence to support its effectiveness?

Intermittent fasting has existed for a long time, and its effectiveness has been studied since then. But in the old days, a very small number of people (usually under 50) were taken as a sample size to experiment, collect data, and analyze. Even though the results favored the effects of intermittent fasting, it nevertheless cannot be used as a generalization.

These results indicate that intermittent fasting provides health benefits other weight loss; studies show that it may help to lower the risk of heart problems and type-2 diabetes in some individuals; however, more research is needed to confirm this.

To do that, large-scale studies are called for. Moreover, other studies have been conducted on animals like rats and monkeys. Some of the claims about the advantages and disadvantages of intermittent fasting are made based on research.

What about longevity?

Longevity is another promise of intermittent fasting because of which it has grown so popular with even well-known celebs incorporating it into their lifestyle. In theory, it does affect lifespan as it slows down the metabolism, repairs and recycles damaged cells. But it's just a claim with limited scientific backing.

Most research on the effects of intermittent fasting on longevity is done on rats. Some rats who were put on intermittent fasting have been reported live 83% longer, which would not be possible for humans. However, even the possibility of living 20% longer evidence would be more than enough to make intermittent fasting more appealing to the masses.

Are there any side effects?

Known long-term or short-term side effects of intermittent fasting are minor. They include headaches, irritation, and fatigue. However, don't stretch yourself too much, too soon. One may develop heartburn, dehydration, and ulcers during the initial days, but your body will adjust accordingly.

Who should not practice intermittent fasting?

Pregnant women, people suffering from eating disorders, people who are chronically stressed, people with injuries who are in the healing phase, and people suffering from life-threatening diseases should not practice intermittent fasting.

CHAPTER

2

Types of Intermittent Fasting Diets

Since the introduction of intermittent fasting, several different variations of this diet have become available for people to follow. Each of these variations has unique benefits that can be gained, as well as considerations for you to think about. They are designed to support you with different goals and assist you in maintaining your best levels of health.

While there are practically countless adaptations of the intermittent fasting diet out there, we are going to focus on just seven in this chapter. Each of these diets adjusts the levels of fasting that you will experience on either a daily or weekly basis. Some will require more fasting than others, whereas some offer more eating time.

Choosing which diet is right for you will depend on a few things. First, you want to consider what you are looking to gain from intermittent fasting. Then, you want to look at which of these adaptations is optimal for achieving those particular goals. You also want to pay attention to any considerations that you may have. If you have any, you will need to make sure that the choice you make is one that accommodates for those considerations. Lastly, you need to choose based on your preference. Determine which one feels as though it will be the best fit for you and start there.

If you decide after some trial and error that the one

you have chosen does not fit your needs or feels too challenging for you to maintain, consider trying a different adaptation. However, make sure that you give each one at least a few weeks' worth of effort to ensure that the challenges you are facing are not simply you getting used to your new diet. Once you have found the one that works for you, simply maintain it, and continue receiving all of the great benefits from it!

2.1
12-Hour Fast

The average person fasts for around eight hours every night. So, the 12-hour fast is not a far stretch from what you likely already naturally do in your everyday life. When you follow the 12-hour fasting diet, you want to maintain equal lengths of fasting and eating windows each day. The easiest way to do this is to eat an earlier supper and a later breakfast.

Completing the 12-hour fast diet should not take too much adjustment to your traditional eating routine. Chances are, you probably already eat pretty close to this type of schedule in your daily life, anyway. The biggest adjustment to this type of fasting is that you truly need to cut out late night snacking. Late night snacking tends to be the primary way that people consume food between 7 PM and 7 AM, anyway. Letting go of this habit can support you in taking on the intermittent fasting eating cycles and gaining many benefits without any drastic changes to your routine.

Another reason why this diet may be easier for beginners is because you still have plenty of time to consume the same number of calories per day that you are used to. Other diets with shorter eating windows typically do not leave enough time for you to get quite as many calories into your day, which can lead to a bit of a transition phase as you get used to your new eating cycles.

The 12-hour fast is a great practice for those who are just starting out with intermittent fasting. Alternatively, it might be a better consideration for those who cannot commit to a more intense variation of the diet for health reasons. Because it does not require any major changes to your present eating routines, it is easy to adapt to and can support you in maintaining any other dietary requirements that you may need to consider.

2.2

16:8 Fasting

The 16:8 fasting diet is similar to the 12-hour fast except that it requires a slightly longer fasting window. This fasting diet can be a little more challenging for some people to adapt to as it requires 16 hours of fasting and only 8 hours of eating. This means that in 8 hours you need to consume any meals and snacks that you want to for the day.

Despite being more intense, the 16:8 diet is still typically an easy one to adjust to. With some minor adjustments to your daily schedule, you can easily accommodate for the longer fasting window. Typically, most people who do the 16:8 diet simply cut out their regular breakfast meal and just focus on lunch and dinner instead. This makes it quite a simple adjustment once you get used to skipping breakfast.

The most common way of eating in alignment with this fast is to stop eating at 8 PM each day and then eat again at 12 noon the next day. This is typically the easiest way to accommodate for the 16 hours of fasting. However, you can also choose to stop eating after dinner and eat an earlier lunch the next day. How you choose to adjust the fasting window is not nearly as important as making sure that you get the full 16 hours of fasting in each day.

For some people, the 16:8 diet may still be quite similar to how they already eat. For both the 12-hour fast and the 16:8 diet, many people find that they instinctively eat this way, to begin with. However, being stricter about not eating during that fasting window can support you in seeing greater health benefits from your dietary habits.

When you are eating in alignment with the 16:8 fasting practice, you see even greater improvements similar to what you see from the 12-hour fast. This makes it a great "step up" for anyone who is not seeing all of the results that they desire to see from the 12-hour fast.

The 16:8 fasting diet is the level of intermittent fasting where many of the most optimal benefits are truly gained. Studies have shown that this variation of the diet is optimal for anyone who is looking to protect against obesity, inflammation, diabetes, and liver disease. These benefits can all be gained even if you continue to consume the same number of calories per day, simply in a shorter window of time. The primary beneficial health factor here is the longer fasting, not the number of calories consumed.

2.3

5:2 Fasting

The original diet to ever be shared and popularized when it came to intermittent fasting was the 5:2 fasting diet. This is a weekly diet, not a daily diet like the previous two we discussed. For the 5:2 fasting diet, you eat as you normally would five days a week and then significantly reduce your calorie intake for two days a week. This ratio is said to support you in gaining all of the benefits of intermittent fasting with relatively little interruption to your regular eating habits.

For the two days that you are fasting, you are still allowed to have a small amount of calorie intake. Typically, men will consume about 600 calories per day and women will consume about 500 calories per day. This gives you enough to refrain from starving, but without interrupting your fast too much.

The most common way to complete the 5:2 diet is to distribute the days throughout the week. Rather than fasting two days in a row, people will fast on one day, eat for three, fast on one day, and eat for two. This ensures that you do not feel as though you are going too long between meals. That way, you maintain your hunger satisfaction and your diet remains sustainable.

For the 5:2 diet, a study was done that showed that more than 100 women who were either overweight or obese lost the same amount of weight using this eating method as they did when restricting calories. However, restricting calories is typically more intense and harder to maintain over time. Many people who restrict calories on a continued basis find themselves struggling to maintain the restriction over time. Furthermore, any time they stop restricting their calories they see more weight gain which can lead to continuous changes in weight. This is not only upsetting to the person dieting but can also be stressful and unhealthy to their body.

2.4
Alternating Days

Alternating which day you fast on is a common variation of the intermittent fasting diet. It also happens to have many of its own unique adaptations. Typically, the one you choose is based on what feels best for you and supports you in getting the best results.

Some people choose to completely avoid any solid foods on their fasting days whereas others will eat up to 500 calories on their fasting days. On days where the individual eats normally, they can eat as much as they want. This is a more intense version of the intermittent fasting diet, and it may take more work to acclimate your body to this dieting habit so that you can maintain it properly. You may also prefer to start with eating up to 500 calories and then reduce to having no solids on your fasting days, or you might just stay with 500 calorie days. For this variation of the diet, the best way to find what works is to play around a bit and see what feels best for you.

Studies have shown that alternating fasting days is effective in supporting individuals with their heart health. It is also an incredible variation for people who want to lose weight. One study that was conducted found that the average person lost about 11 pounds over a 12 week period using this diet.

Because of how extreme this fasting diet can be, it is not ideal for anyone who has never fasted before. Even if you have naturally fasted for fairly extended periods of time, you should first work towards intentionally sustaining a more relaxed variation of the intermittent fasting diet before moving to alternating days. You should also avoid this fasting style if you are dealing with certain medical conditions as it can have a negative impact on you. If you are considering the alternating days diet for intermittent fasting, be sure to let your doctor know your specific plans. This can help them determine what would be the right decision for you to make so that you don't face any adverse health repercussions.

2.5
24 Hour Weekly Fasting

Similar to the 5:2 fast is the 24-hour weekly fast. This variation of the diet allows people to consume food normally six days per week, and then completely fast for 24 hours. During this 24 hour window, absolutely no food should be consumed. Individuals are also encouraged to avoid drinking any drinks that may be too high in calories, such as whole milk lattés or smoothies.

This variation of the diet is often called the "eat-stop-eat" diet because it only requires one day of true change on a weekly basis. Otherwise, you can eat whatever you want and however you want. For those who are seeking to incorporate weekly dieting into their eating plans, the 24-hour weekly fast is a great place to start. This is a relatively relaxed place to start. For some people, it may offer plenty enough benefits to make it a good place to stay, too. For others, they may prefer to adjust to the 5:2 diet after they get used to it so that they can see greater results from their efforts.

It is important to be cautious of how the 24-hour weekly fast impacts you. While some people find great success with this, other people find that one single day per week is not frequently enough so their body never fully acclimates. As a result, they end up experiencing headaches, fatigue, or even irritability during their fasting day. For most, these symptoms outweigh the benefits that they gain, which results in them not maintaining the 24-hour fasting cycle. If you still want to give this eating pattern a try, you may benefit from first using the 16:8 fasting method before adjusting to test out the 24-hour weekly fasting. This can support your body with getting used to the changes.

2.6
Meal Skipping

Meal skipping is an extremely flexible form of intermittent fasting that can provide all of the benefits of intermittent fasting but with less of the strict scheduling. If you are not someone who has a typical schedule or who feels as though a stricter variation of the intermittent fasting diet will serve you, meal skipping is a viable alternative.

Many people who choose to use meal skipping find it to be a great way to listen to their body and follow their basic instincts. If they are not hungry, they simply don't eat that meal. Instead, they wait for the next one. Meal skipping can also be helpful for people who have time constraints and who may not always be able to get in a certain meal of the day.

The best way to make meal skipping successful is to learn how to stay in tune with your body and focus on what it needs. Often, people discover that they simply don't become hungry 3+ times per day. So, instead of eating several meals, they only eat when they are hungry.

It is important to realize that with meal skipping, you may not always be maintaining a 10-16 hour window of fasting. As a result, you may not get every benefit that comes from other fasting diets. However, this may be a great solution to people who want an intermittent fasting diet that feels more natural to them. It may also be a great idea for those who are looking to begin listening to their body more so that they can adjust to a more intense variation of the diet with greater ease. In other words, it can be a great transitional diet for you if you are not ready to jump into one of the other fasting diets just yet.

2.7

Warrior Diet Fasting

The most extreme form of intermittent fasting is known as the Warrior Diet. This intermittent fasting cycle follows a 20-hour fasting window with a short 4-hour eating window. During that eating window, individuals are supposed to only consume raw fruits and vegetables. They can also eat one large meal. Typically, the eating window takes place at night time so people can snack throughout the evening, have a large meal, and then resume fasting.

Because of the length of fasting taking place during

the Warrior Diet, people should also consume a fairly hearty level of healthy fats. Doing so will give the body something to consume during the fast to produce energy with. A small amount of carbohydrates can also be incorporated to support energy levels, too.

People who eat the Warrior Diet tend to believe that humans are natural nocturnal eaters and that we are not meant to eat throughout the day. The belief is that eating this way follows our natural circadian rhythms, allowing our body to work optimally.

The only people who should consider doing the Warrior Diet are those who have already had success with other forms of intermittent fasting and who are used to it. Attempting to jump straight into the Warrior Diet can have serious repercussions for anyone who is not used to intermittent fasting. Even still, those who are used to it may find this particular style to be too extreme for them to maintain.

It is important that if you do work up to the Warrior Diet that you stay very vigilant over your personal health. If you are not careful, you might find that you become malnourished or that you struggle with other health issues. These health issues are counterintuitive and actually increase your risk of contracting illnesses like cancer, rather than decrease it.

Still, those who have learned to eat according to the Warrior Diet ways and who have acclimated to it say they feel as though they are in optimal health. They tend to have great energy levels, minimal fat stores, and healthier systems overall. That is, if they are maintaining their nourishment within that 4-hour eating window. Those who are have not experienced great success with this diet and often find themselves struggling to maintain it.

CHAPTER

3

The Best Food Types and Optimal Meal Plans for Intermittent Fasting

In order for intermittent fasting to work as a whole, there is no restriction on what you can or cannot eat.

However, if you aren't eating the right foods while you are eating, then you won't get the results that you want. You might lose a couple of pounds, but to see a significant reduction, you should ensure that you are eating the best foods and stick to an optimal meal plan. Intermittent fasting itself isn't its own diet. Instead, it's more of an accessory to help make your chosen meal plan work even better.

Throughout this chapter, we are going to discuss the best possible foods that you can include in your diet. I don't think I need to mention again the risk of highly sugary foods, so we won't talk about what to avoid anymore. Instead, let's take a look at not just which foods are best for you overall, but which meal plans might work with your diet as well.

Best Food Types

The best thing for you that you can consume as much as you want, whenever you want as long as it's water. Water makes up a big part of most living things in the world, and all food that is healthy to be eaten has been alive at one point, such as plants and animals.

Salt, honey, alcohol, artificial sweeteners and additives,

eggs, and dairy products weren't alive, but some of these should be avoided in your diet anyway. Healthy dairy products will have live cultures in them as well. Anyway, that's not the point. The point is, you need to include a ton of water while fasting and while not.

When you're fasting, the water will keep things moving. Some people will find that they suffer from constipation during a fast because they aren't drinking enough water. While you're eating, pairing water with everything will help fill in the spaces and make you feel fuller.

Always have water as a side drink for other things. So, if you choose to indulge in a soda, or have a beer or a glass of wine with dinner, pair it with water. Take two sips of water for every one sip of something else that you drink.

Water can be boring, but it doesn't have to be the main show! It's just something that you need to have all the time to help your body. It's like the best medicine possible for a ton of minor conditions, such as heartburn, headache, being tired, and other small things. There's nothing that a glass of water can't help at least make feel better. We have water dishes out for our pets all day, so you should have a water bottle by your side. If you can carry your phone with you everywhere you go, then you can carry a small bottle of water as well. There are no excuses not to be drinking enough water unless of course, you don't have access to clean drinking water, so make sure to have this as a huge part of your diet.

Moving on, whole grains are going to be an important addition to your diet. Many people will become fearful of carbohydrates, and they are avoided in some diets, such as a ketogenic diet. However, carbohydrates are dangerous when they come from refined sugars. Carbs are really our main source of energy, so it's important that they are considered in your diet.

Whole grains contain fiber, protein, and other important vitamins and minerals that will provide your body with some of the best things that it needs for proper function. What you need to put an emphasis on when choosing carbs is that they are whole grains, and state that they are %100 whole wheat and not white carbs like bread and pasta.

The reason for this is because these white carbs are stripped of the things that make them actually good for you. The whole wheat is actually stripped down and left with just the tasty part; the health benefits being gone. This means that these white carbs are easily broken-down sugars, making them more likely to be stored as fat.

Whole wheat takes a bit longer for your body to process and will provide more energy for longer periods of time throughout the day, making them especially helpful for starting a fast. You might be tempted to jump right into a diet like a keto diet in order to shed pounds but starting a fast with whole grains on your eating days might help to curb your appetite a bit.

Moving onto our proteins, always choose things that are lean meats and rich in omega-3 fatty acids. Healthy protein is important because it provides us with the healthy kinds of fats our body needs to function.

A lot of meat that you will find in stores is highly processed as well. For example, chicken and turkey should have almost 0 carbs per serving, and sometimes you might see < 1g labeled as the amount for a serving just for the company to cover their bases. For the most part, it should be 0. However, if you go up to any deli section and look at the nutrition facts on some meat, they will say 3g or more per serving, meaning that they are processed and contain added sugars.

When choosing meats like chicken and beef, you want to look for food that is grass-fed, organic, or free range. The biggest meat producers will give their animals just what they need to survive, often fed with grains. While this isn't going to prevent you from losing a ton of weight versus other foods you might decide to eat, it's still something that should be considered for your health, as you want protein which contains omega-3 fatty acids.

Fruits and veggies are given in terms of choosing to eat these over anything else. Just ensure that you aren't loading them up with other sneaky carbs and sugars, like salad dressings, dips, and hummus. These things aren't always bad, but store-bought might contain sneaky salts and sugars that make them just as unhealthy as other junky snacks.

Look for ways that vegetables can replace some other unhealthy things, like white pasta, in your diet. You might consider using lettuce as a wrap or a bun for a burger versus white bread. You might use zucchini noodles instead of white pasta noodles.

Whatever it is that you choose, as long as you're focusing on adding more veggies and less of everything else, you're starting off with the right decisions.

Also consider adding dark leafy greens to your diet, as these will be among the best veggies. Spinach and kale are good choices to add to any salad over iceberg lettuce, as they are packed with essential nutrition than some other water lettuce.

As far as fruit goes, make sure you still eat this in moderation as even though it's natural, it does have more sugar. A handful of strawberries is always better than a handful of chocolate. You can even blend fruit together with a little milk to get a tasty smoothie – a great sweet treat.

When picking fruits, go for berries first. These are rich with antioxidants, which can help keep your immune system in check and provide you with important anti-inflammatory properties.

Aside from grains, fruits, veggies, and meat, make sure to choose the right kind of dairy as well. Avoid processed cheeses like you would meats and go for things that are more natural. Flavored sweet dairy products, like yogurt, should be eaten in moderation. Plain Greek yogurt can be great for you and could be used as a mayonnaise alternative, especially in things like chicken salad. Skim milk is a good choice for cereals, pasta sauces, and gravies. Choosing non-dairy milk, like soy or almond, is a great decision as well, and can provide you with an extra source of protein.

When you're fasting, on the days when you might eat, you should look for alternate protein methods, such as black beans and tofu. Not only is this healthier for you, but it can have added benefits to the environment when we cut down on our meat intake.

Optimal Meal Plans for Intermittent Fasting

This book is just about fasting, but it's still important to include some ideas for meal plans that you might see. You might often see fasting regimens paired with a ketogenic diet. Some other healthy alternatives might be the Mediterranean diet, as well as the DASH diet.

In order to pick a meal plan, think of what goals you might have. Do you want to lose 100 pounds? Do you want to reduce your risk of cancer? Do you want to regulate your cardiovascular system?

All of these diets have been shown to have improvements in all of these areas, but let's look at them a bit further to determine one that might be right for you. Of course, everyone should do their best to eat healthy foods as we described above, but to get more specific results, you can choose from popular meal plans.

The most popular diet you will see with intermittent fasting, and one popular among celebrities and other notable fitness influencers is the ketogenic diet. What is included in this is a diet focused on cutting out carbohydrates, specifically to less than around 50 grams (depending on an individual's biology). The main source of energy would then come from fat, both on your body and healthy fats that are added to your diet.

The point of this is to cause your body to burn even more fat. Your body currently uses carbohydrates as the main source of energy. When you take that away, your body will still need energy, so it will look elsewhere.

Some don't think that keto diets are as healthy because it requires you to include more fat in your diet, making some think it's bad for your heart. The goal, however, should be to include healthy fats, through things like avocados, salmon, and other types of fish, rather than through fats like bacon, cream cheese, and a spoonful of coconut oil. If you want to lose a larger amount of weight in a faster time period, consider this diet.

One diet that seems to bring on a plethora of health benefits is the Mediterranean diet. This is based on diets eaten in countries which surround the Mediterranean Sea like Spain, Italy, Greece, Turkey, Egypt, Morocco, and so on.

This diet is popular because scientific studies show that the people who live here have a longer life expectancy and less chance of cancer and other types of health conditions. The food involved in a Mediterranean diet includes whole grains, legumes, and plenty of fruits and veggies. Red meat, and most meat in general is eaten less than once a month, and most dairy is cut out, aside from the occasional feta. This diet is considered one of the healthiest in the world, which is why it can be a good choice for those looking for longevity and reduced risk of other health conditions.

Finally, another popular diet for you to consider is the DASH diet. This stands for Dietary Approaches to Stop Hypertension. This diet has been around for decades and was created in order to reduce heart disease, as hypertension affects almost a billion people all across the world (National Institutes of Health, 2018).

The DASH diet is mainly focused on including grains, veggies, fruits, dairy products, meats, nuts, and fats/oils. It is most commonly visualized using a plate, with the grain and veggie portions being the biggest. It is an easier diet that would be a good place to start if you're not sure where to begin with your healthy eating plans.

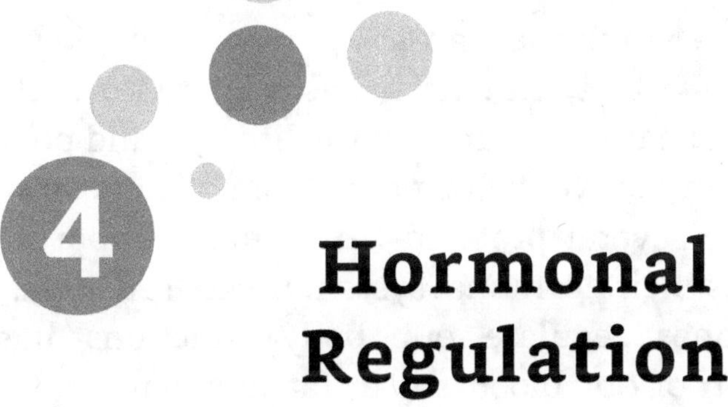

4 Hormonal Regulation

Hormones are important. The way your body functions has a lot to do with your hormonal health. Bad and erratic lifestyle and poor food choices can toss your hormonal balance for a spin. This can cause several problems. It is more important for women as their hormonal system is very sensitive.

Hormones regulate our body functions like the regulation of our blood sugar, fat metabolism, hunger, and satiety all. Intermittent fasting can play a very important role in regulating these hormones so that you can achieve optimal health and lose weight.

Impact of Intermittent Fasting on Various Hormones: Insulin

We have already discussed that insulin is an important hormone that balances your blood sugar levels and also causes fat storage. If the amount of insulin present in your bloodstream remains consistently high, it will inhibit any kind of fat loss. However, it will also cause another serious problem called insulin resistance. It is a condition in which your body stops responding well to the insulin released by the pancreas. It may not sound scary as such, but this is the condition which leads to diabetes later on.

Intermittent fasting helps your body by regulating the presence of insulin in the body. The long interval between the meals ensures that your bloodstream has a lower concentration of insulin. The prolonged absence of the hormone helps you cells in becoming more receptive to the hormone. In this way, intermittent fasting helps you in developing insulin sensitivity which is one of the most positive steps toward good health. We will be discussing this aspect in detail in the chapter discussing the impact of intermittent fasting on diabetes.

Human Growth Hormone

This is also a hormone that helps in fat burning. We have discussed in detail the impact intermittent fasting has on the production of growth hormone. Higher the amount of growth hormone production in your body, the better will be your fat burning, muscle growth, immunity, recovery, etc. It is a very important hormone that has gained great curiosity in the professional bodybuilding community and among athletes. The reason is simple; this hormone can help in gaining muscles much faster than anything else and also improves your endurance.

This hormone has received a lot of flak around the world as people have started misusing the synthetic form of the growth hormone for increasing their performance. It is not only illegal to use it, but it is highly dangerous too. The artificially produced growth hormone may have a similar molecular structure to the natural one but it isn't the same, and therefore, it can have a very negative impact on the health of an individual. It is a reason the use of this hormone has been banned globally.

Intermittent fasting, on the other hand, helps you in producing large amounts of growth hormones naturally. This not only boosts fat burning but also helps you in gaining muscle strength. The production of growth hormone is the highest when you exercise on an empty stomach at the end of your intermittent fast. It produces a very strong fat burning effect on your body.

Cortisol

The purpose is to aid your body in its work.

So, if you are constantly eating while the stress hormones in your body are high, it will start helping in the accumulation of fat. This is a reason people who are going through depression, diseases or low phases in their lives gain so much weight. However, if you are following intermittent fasting, it will give your stress hormones a signal that your body is trying to burn the fat. These hormones will then start helping in burning the fat. Intermittent fasting also helps in reducing the levels of stress hormones in your body, and therefore you can eventually get rid of rapid weight gain or loss effect.

Adrenaline

This is also a stress hormone that is released by your adrenal glands. However, the interesting thing to note is the impact adrenaline hormone has on fat burning and muscle building. This hormone increases your ability to do exercise and builds your stamina. Intermittent fasting can help in increasing the production of this hormone along with the growth hormone as the conditions for the production of both these hormones are the same.

Ghrelin

This is the hunger hormone. Your gut produces this hormone to send a signal to your brain to make you eat something. This hormone has several other functions too besides inducing hunger like it also aids the production of the growth hormone and the adrenaline. It also aids the production of several hormones that affect fertility and ovulation in women. However, the main function of this hormone is to make your brain know that you need to eat something.

The release of ghrelin hormone should be at its peak when your stomach is empty, and it starts receding as you eat. The levels of ghrelin are the lowest after 20 minutes of your finishing the meal. It signals that you do not need to eat anymore.

However, frequent intake of food can have a very bad effect on your gut. It gets overworked and doesn't get time to recover. Fast food, processed food, and food with high quantities of unhealthy things can also cause chronic inflammation too in your gut. The inflammation in your gut can mess up with the release of this hormone. Your gut can start releasing ghrelin in moderate quantities all the time. This will confuse your brain, and you will never be able to identify real hunger. This can make you feel tempted to food all the time.

Intermittent fasting coupled with the right kind of food can help you in regularizing the ghrelin hormone release. First, controlled periods of feasting and fasting give your gut the time to process the consumed food properly. Your gut will be able to digest things properly and will not have to push food in the intestines due to want of space. This will help in curing chronic inflammation.

Second, anti-inflammatory food and food with high fiber content has a soothing impact. The food with high fiber content takes very long to get digested while it releases very small amounts of energy. This keeps you feeling fuller for longer without stuffing you with calories. It also helps in regulating your ghrelin release as your gut will not release ghrelin till there is food inside it. This helps in making your brain more sensitive to ghrelin release.

Leptin

This is the satiety hormone. It means that the job of this hormone is to instruct your brain to stop eating when your fat reserves are full. This hormone is released by your fat cells in the adipose tissues. The higher the amount of fat in your body, the greater is the release of leptin. It means, ideally obese people should feel less hungry as their fat deposits are already high. However, that doesn't happen in the real world.

In fact, the people who are obese generally find it difficult to suppress their hunger. The reason is the unregulated release of leptin hormone and the subsequent leptin resistance developed by the brain which makes it insensitive to the signals.

When you start eating something, the release of leptin should be the lowest, and it should peak around the time when you have eaten your fill. This difference in the leptin levels will make the hypothalamus of your brain recognize the signal, and it will instruct you to stop eating. However, when there is chronic inflammation in the fat cells, they keep releasing the leptin hormone at all times. It means neither the excretion of the hormone is very low when you are hungry, nor it is very high when you are full. It is always almost the same. This confuses the brain as it is not able to decipher the meaning of the signal. Hence, obese people will never really feel satiated. They are not eating out of the need for food, but they eat due to their inability to feel satiety.

Intermittent fasting can help in this situation in many ways. First, intermittent fasting has a very positive impact on chronic inflammations in your body.

Second, intermittent fasting leads to the creation of temporary feasting and fasting periods. During the fasting gaps, your body is forced to burn the stored fat. This creates an actual need for energy. Your leptin levels really go down when your body is burning fat. This creates a difference between the leptin levels in your blood during fasting and feasting. This difference helps in making your brain more sensitive to the signals. While practicing intermittent fasting, you will be able to feel actual satiety while eating.

Third, intermittent fasting helps in reducing the amount of free fatty acids in your blood as they are used for producing energy. These free fatty acids otherwise interfere with the leptin signaling. Hence, you can have better leptin sensitivity.

Therefore;

You can see that intermittent fasting can have a very robust impact on hormonal regulation. It can help you in staying healthy and fit. However, before you move ahead, women need to take this information with a pinch of salt.

Although intermittent fasting can help in regulating all these hormones, the body of women can react in a pretty harsh way to these changes. Change is good, but a drastic change can have an adverse effect. In order to remain on the safe side, it is important that women should use caution while following intermittent fasting.

The Good, the Bad, and the Ugly

When it comes female hormonal system there really is a good, bad, and the ugly side of it. To begin with, it is super sensitive. This means that red flags can rise even when nothing significant takes place.

The body of a woman can react in a very quick way to fasting, and it can also react harshly. That is why women are never advised to change their lifestyle abruptly.

You must always start by making moderate changes in your lifestyle. If you want to keep 14 hours fasts in a day as it gives great results. You must never start with 14 hours at first. You must always begin with cutting the snacks from your routines first. Then try to put a proper gap between the three meals in a day. Slowly move ahead to fasting for 12 hours in a day and eating for the remaining 12.

Keeping the fasts on two non-consecutive days of a week also works fine for women as their bodies find it less taxing.

Whatever, the way you choose to do this, it is important that you do not throw your body out of balance. Your hormonal system is delicate and starving yourself all of a sudden can activate binge eating. That way you will end up consuming more calories than required. Keeping yourself hungry for long can also cause mood swings and irritability.

The fertility of women who forcibly starve themselves for too long also gets affected.

It is again important to reiterate the fact that intermittent fasting is a long-term lifestyle change that brings beneficial results. Jumping on to a tough regimen will not only send you on a hunger drive but will also wreck your hormones.

The ghrelin and leptin balance is the first to get affected. However, it is important to understand here that it mostly becomes a problem for lean women who are trying to manage their weight at a certain level. If you are overweight, your fertility and ovulation cycles won't get affected much as the fat levels in your body will be very high and hence real starvation will not be kicking in anytime soon.

Yet, all women should follow moderation while practicing intermittent fasting. Several intermittent fasting protocols can be followed as per the need and endurance of your body. All intermittent fasting protocols have their own specific advantages, and hence it would be hasty to believe that any tougher regimen would bring better results much faster. Only a healthy change will bring the best results when it comes to intermittent fasting.

You must always keep this in mind and never take up any longer fast without getting habitual to similar fast of lower intensity.

If practiced properly, intermittent fasting can help you in achieving a great hormonal balance. You will feel more energized and recharged. There will be no lack of energy or enthusiasm. You will feel more content and happy.

You will be able to enjoy almost all kinds of food that you like and still remain in shape. Hormonal regulation also has a very strong impact on your psychological health apart from physiological health. You will experience a drastic change in your attitude as it will become more positive and accepting.

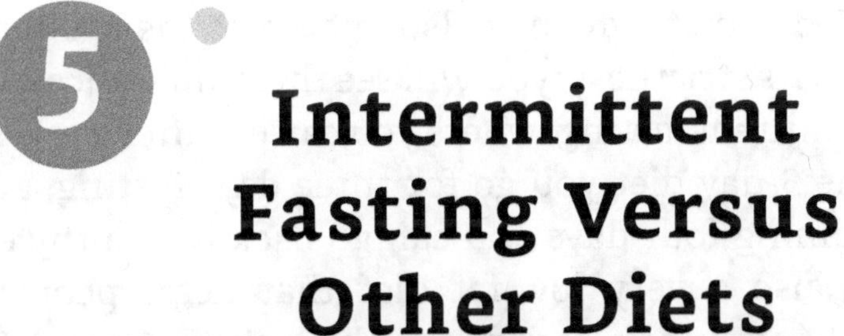

5 Intermittent Fasting Versus Other Diets

Any diet that makes someone go without food for some time is known as I intermittent fasting. When you compare intermittent fasting with the 3-day diet, which is also known as the military diet due to its strictness, you will see their differences. Unlike intermittent fasting, where you can eat after a few hours, in the 3-day diet you go for three days fasting, and the remaining four days you can go back to healthy eating. It is also a very low-fat diet that helps people shed weight extremely fast due to the lack of calories. Unlike intermittent fasting, with the 3-day fasting, calories will come back full force when the calorie period is over. It also does not provide the nutrients needed by the body because of the intake of the required amount of fruits and vegetables is strictly limited, unlike in intermittent fasting.

A master cleanse lemonade diet is also another diet plan that helps in weight loss. Unlike the intermittent where you can have meals at stipulated times, the master cleanses lemonade diet only allows you to drink a beverage that resembles lemonade and salt water through the ten days. Intermittent fasting has significant health benefits, but the same cannot be said for the masters cleanse lemonade diet. This is because, during the ten days, you will not take the required number of calories or nutrients that boost the immunity of the body, and the calorie intake is restricted to 650 only. Unlike in the intermittent fasting diet where your cravings and eating habits may be improved, in the master cleanse diet, you may end up overeating after the diet plan and gain even more weight.

Fast diet is different from intermittent fasting in that a person is not allowed to have a heavy meal during the eating window. That is why some people find it hard to follow religiously. With the fast day diet, it is almost impossible to get your daily required nutrients. That is because even calorie intake is supposed to be less than 500 in women and less than 600 in men that will only meet your daily energy limit. The good thing about intermittent fasting is that during the eating window, you do not have to count the calories you consume, making it a preferable diet. Studies carried out suggested that unlike the fast meal plan, intermittent fasting increased longevity in both men and women and had more health benefits.

5.1

Intermittent fasting shopping list

For the first three days of fasting, you will need to shop for the following food items.

Fish

It is essential to include fish in your shopping list. This is because it usually contains healthy fats and proteins the right amount of vitamin D. Your meals should be packed with more nutrients. They will help your body and fish will ensure you get them, including feeding your brain.

Potatoes

Potatoes are one of the best foods in making someone full. This is because it takes minimum effort for the body to digest. During intermittent fasting, vegetables are essential, especially when cooled it forms a starch primed resistance which helps in fueling good bacteria found in the gut.

Berries

Vitamin C, which is used in the boosting of the immune system, is found in strawberries. Studies suggest that when added to your intermittent fasting diet, it can help in the reduction of your body mass index over 14 years. This is thanks to vital nutrients such as flavonoids.

Nuts

Nuts have been known to remove body fat and help in longevity and reduce the risk of cardiovascular illnesses such as type 2 diabetes. The presence of polyunsaturated fats in nuts can help a person to feel fuller for long hours.

Eggs

Eggs usually contain proteins which are essential during intermittent fasting as it will keep the body full for longer hours and help in the building of muscles. A study that was carried out showed that when some men ate a bagel for breakfast, they tended to be more hungry than their counterparts that fed on eggs for breakfast. This made them feed on more calories throughout the day, causing them to lose very minimal weight.

Whole grains

Whole grains are one of the items that should be included in your shopping list when doing intermittent fasting. This is because they contain vibrant levels of protein and fiber, making a person feel full for long hours. Whole grains like lentils are perfect when it comes to iron, which is very important, especially for women who are fasting.

Salmon

Salmon is another critical item to include on your intermittent fasting shopping list because of its links with longevity. Salmon also has high levels of EPA and DHA, which are the omega-three fatty acids that boost the brain functions.

Fortified vitamin D milk

Fortified vitamin D milk is vital because it highly increases the capability of the body to absorb calcium. The calcium helps the bones, and the good thing is that you can use it in your cereals or even smoothies.

Pawpaw

Pawpaw is one of the critical items that you have to include in your shopping list. This is because it contains essential enzymes known as papain that are usually used to break down proteins. These enzymes help reducing issues caused by overeating such as bloating, especially when you just started intermittent fasting and you go for hours without eating.

Water

Water is one of the essential items on the list because it helps you stay hydrated for the excellent health and optimum function of almost all organs in the body. Dehydration causes fatigue and lightheadedness. You will expel dark yellow urine, which is very smelly, and when you can go through this with unlimited food, it can be hazardous.

5.2

Intermittent fasting meal plan

Intermittent fasting can be used as a weight-loss tool, and above all, it has very many health benefits. Below is an intermittent fasting meal plan that will see to it that you have a smooth fast.

9 am- black tea

When doing the intermittent fasting, most of your eating habits will change, and this is because you will have to accommodate healthier meals and beverages. Taking black tea is healthy because it is a calorie-free drink.

11 am -1.30pm mild workout and lots of water

At this time, you are required to drink lots of water and stay busy. When you remain idle, it is very easy, falling into temptation and binge eating is very easy. Try and be as active as you can be. Mild exercises such as walking, doing house chores that keep you busy until your eating window. Being proactive will help your mind to be more alert.

2pm-3.30 pm drink sparkling water

When you are almost finishing your fast, and you have a strong urge to have something more than water in your tummy. You can go for sparkling water. It usually has zero calories and makes one feel fuller for longer. This is advantageous because when you feel full, you will not crave for unhealthy meals.

4 pm breaking of the fast

You can use a low-calorie protein bar and a fruit to break your fast. Apples are the most preferred fruit for breaking a fast as they low in calorie, and the larger capacity is water. Apples are also very palatable and make someone stay fuller for longer, and the good news is it contains minimal calories. Apple also have carbohydrates that

4.30 pm – 7 pm

When you snack in the afternoon, your body may start to feel hungrier. The calorie intake for the afternoon snack should be less than 500 calories. All you need to do is be patient to let the food you ate before to start providing energy for the body. You do not have to take more snacks, be active, and try not to think about the hunger so much. Try and run some errands or work on some projects as you wait for the energy to start being produced.

7.30pm meal time

At this time, you can now pay yourself off by having one hearty meal. You are allowed to have a substantial amount of food. The meal is supposed to be your primary calorie source, so this means that you have to eat a well-balanced meal. You are not only supposed to have a big meal but to also make sure there is a right balance of macronutrients. The level of proteins should be higher than fat and carbohydrates, which should be taken in moderation. Every meal should at least contain less than 1000 calories. Some of the foods you can take during a meal are rice, white meat either fish of skinned chicken, vegetables, and some cheese which will provide fat content in the feed. Another simple, quick meal that you can consume during your eating period is pasta, minced meat with some vegetables of your choice. When you decide to go out for dinner, you can always order food that has the same nutrients as the ones discussed above but still try and eat moderately.

At 11 pm you can have your dessert

After your meal, you can have one last dessert before going to bed. Your last snack should be high in protein, but less than 400 calories, and this is dependent on the number of calories you have had during the day.

This works like magic every time you fast. It is ok to try your recipes as long as they are healthy. If they contain all the required nutrients, you are good to go. You should at least try and not go above 2000 calories per day because it might be too much.

Some people might choose to bulk when doing intermittent fasting. Bulking has benefits such as increased human growth hormones that help with the growth of muscles. It can also increase insulin sensitivity, which will, in turn, make your gains leaner. Recent studies concluded that when you lose weight, you can easily preserve your muscle mass. When bulking, your body will need more calories than the one found in the meal plan shown above, so in that case, all you need to do is add more calories. Foods that will help with this are oatmeal, Greek yogurt, and at times, cheese quesadilla.

5.3
Frequently asked questions

How will intermittent fasting slow down aging?

Intermittent fasting has been proved to help people from the risks of cardiovascular diseases. These and other conditions or risk factors that are age-related like Alzheimer's disease by lowering the inflation in the brain protecting the nerve cells is also a benefit of intermittent fasting. Studies that were carried out on animals showed that intermittent fasting activated autophagy that is the process of the cells in the body breaks down dysfunctional cells. It helps in the secretion of the human growth hormones that boost the process of burning fat.

Is it ok to exercise while fasting?

For beginners, it is advisable to exercise less because the body does not have enough energy. A study showed that those who did exercise while fasting lost more weight than those who did not. When your fasting window is at night, then a morning exercise before breakfast is advisable. This is because then, your body will burn more fat due to the depletion of glycogen.

Is intermittent fasting safe?

Many people have benefited from practicing intermittent fasting, especially the shorter ones which are less than 24 hours. This, however, does not mean that it is safe for everyone. Pregnant women, children, and people who have type 1 diabetes are not advised to fast.

What is intermittent fasting?

Intermittent fasting is the use of cycles to fast and eat to lose weight and for other health benefits such as cardiovascular health. Studies have shown that intermittent fasting can help in the reduction of chronic illnesses such as diabetes type 2. Other diseases are hypertension and even diseases that affect the brain negatively, such as Alzheimer's disease.

Is it ok to take supplements during fasting?

Taking supplements when fasting is ok when fasting.

How many types of intermittent fasting do we have?

There are many different types of intermittent fasting, but the most common ones are the 12-hour fasting and 12-hour eating window. This is the most advised fasting method for beginners. The 16/8 way is another method that involves fasting for 16 hours in a day and restricting your eating for the remaining 8 hours. There is also the 5:2 diet. It is the method whereby you limit your calorie intake to 600 maximum on two days of the week, which does not have to be consecutive. Then the other standard way is the 24-hour fasting whereby you go for a whole day without eating. For example, when you eat supper today, you wait up to the next day from you to eat.

Can intermittent fasting help a diabetic person?

Research has shown that intermittent fasting can help in the reduction of suffering from diabetes type 2.

That is because fasting will lower blood sugar levels and reduce insulin resistance.

Does fasting affect your hormones?

Intermittent fasting can positively affect your hormones because during a fast, the level of hormones such as the human growth hormones improved by almost five times. It also causes the cells to repair themselves, thus removing the old ones that are not functioning well and replacing them with ones that work correctly.

6

Six Techniques for Intermittent Fasting

At its core, an intermittent fast is simply the strategy of not eating for one period before eating again for a set period. Within this framework, there are several ways to set your fasting schedule, depending on your goals and your current health conditions—and as a woman, some techniques are more favorable than others.

It is important to note that for any of the following methods to be effective, you must be choosing healthy foods as much as possible for every calorie consumed during your eating window—and remember, everything you drink is considered a calorie as well! Hence, diet sodas, fruit smoothies, and other beverages that disguise themselves as healthy drinks will have an impact on the effectiveness of your plan—if you are disciplined enough to abstain from eating during a time frame, use that same self-control to eliminate junk food and reach for water, tea, or black coffee instead. When you stick with the program, you will find a renewed source of energy and will no longer feel the need for a 'pick me up' from sugar and caffeine.

Meal Skipping

This technique is not technically a fast, but if you are

nervous about jumping into intermittent fasting right away, you could tiptoe in by selecting one meal per day that you will skip, depending on the level of hunger. The main benefit of this approach is to get you accustomed to your body's reaction. For this introduction to be successful, it is important to be mindful of your body's signals and not give in to the first sign of hunger. When you think you feel hunger, typically around lunch, evaluate that feeling, acknowledge what it is, and encourage yourself to carry on a bit longer without giving in to the urge. When you feel what you perceive as hunger, ask yourself, "Have I drunk water today?" When your body tells you, "I'm hungry," what it is often trying to say is, "I'm dehydrated." When you feel hunger pangs, reach for a glass of water first and let that take the edge off. Evaluate yourself after approximately 30 minutes and see if you can carry on with your day until dinner—and each time you think you feel hunger, reach for water again. You will be surprised at how effective this is in keeping the hunger thoughts under control.

This flexible plan can help you by reducing the overall calories in a day which can provide mild benefits if the goal is weight loss however to realize the full benefits of intermittent fasting the body needs to have 8 - 12 hours between meals to enter into the fat-burning metabolic state that triggers all the incredible systems within your body to access energy stores and rewire neural pathways. If you skip lunch but still snack late into the night, you won't be creating the environment needed to enter a fasted state and may run the risk of your body turning to energy sources found in muscle versus the valuable sources found in fat.

If your goal is to begin experimenting with fasting and loss a small amount of weight, meal skipping could be an option, to begin with, but only as a stepping stone to a more structured fasting plan.

The 12-Hour Fasting Technique (12:12)

The 12:12 technique is the ideal fast for beginners, as the fasting window can be planned for your sleeping hours so that the window of time to avoid eating can be a dream! On this plan, you will choose an eating window that suits your life the best. If you are an early riser and want to eat breakfast, you can set your eating window for 6am to 6pm—or if you know that your work schedule means you eat dinner later, you can set your eating window for 8am to 8pm to accommodate. This is a flexible plan that allows you to set the schedule based on your circumstances and can even be adjusted day to day if you prefer ultimate flexibility.

This technique provides that 8-12-hour window needed after eating for the body to digest, absorb, and then begin searching for the stored energy to burn off, otherwise known as being in a fasted state. The key to the fasting window is to stop eating on time and at the end of your last meal. The main culprit to any nutrition plan is going to be late-night snacking so by setting the goal to stop consuming all calories - this means beverages too - at a certain point you will have an immediate impact on calorie reduction which on its own will lead to at a minimum, weight loss, and by adhering to a time frame that creates a fasted state you can begin to enjoy some of the many more subtle benefits of fasting such as reduced inflammation, improved cognitive function, and cellular regeneration.

It should be noted that if you are also a beginner to eating whole foods and healthier options you may find the hunger signals in the morning to be very strong, especially if your body is used to a dose of carbohydrates and processed meats, fats and sugars. This would be your typical drive-thru breakfast combo or even something that disguises itself as a health food, like prepackaged oatmeal in fun flavors like maple pecan, muffins or breakfast cereals. These foods are empty calories and do not provide the nutrients needed to thrive. You have to start looking at every bite as a source of fuel, and when you can recognize a balanced meal with carbohydrates and fiber from whole grains, fruits, and vegetables, protein from plants or animal sources and healthy fats from foods such as avocado, healthy oils or nuts and seeds, you will be providing your body with what it needs to function properly, you will feel fuller for longer periods of time and you will begin to notice the hunger sensations decrease as your body is satiated by nutrient-dense foods.

The 16-Hour (for Men) or the 14-Hour (for Women) Technique (16:8)

This technique stretches the fasting window to either 14 hours or 16 hours, and it is typically scheduled from 12pm to 8pm (if you follow the 16 hours) or 10am to 8pm (if you follow the 14 hours). The window is slightly longer than the 12:12 method, which provides the body with more time in the fasted state to use up stored energy before providing the first dose of readily available nutrition through the macronutrients in your first meal. This fasting schedule can be followed 7 days a week or only as frequently as you see fit. As a beginner, you can choose to follow this schedule for a few days a week as you track and monitor your body's response, or you may decide to jump right in and follow the schedule for the entire week, or perhaps just Monday to Friday and leave the weekends to be more flexible. This flexibility is one of the benefits of intermittent fasting as opposed to a diet based on approved foods or capped calorie amounts—being able to mold the framework of your nutrition plan to suit your specific needs brings certain freedom to your daily life.

As a woman entering the world of intermittent fasting, it is important to take things slowly and listen to the signals your body is providing. Every person will react slightly different to a fast given a number of circumstances such as existing energy stores, your current health conditions, the state of your hormonal balance, and whether you are eating healthy, unprocessed foods already or if you need to also transition your body off the imbalances caused by a poor diet. For women, the changes to metabolic states and the cascading effects on the hormones that regulate menstruation and fertility can be severe and may cause changes to your menstrual cycle. In some cases of severe fasting, women may find they skip their period entirely, which is not a healthy side effect of a healthy diet. Your period is a vital component to your health, and any significant changes to it can indicate larger issues that you will want to address. If you are planning a family and need a healthy regular cycle, be cautious about beginning any sort of fast until you have a solid understanding of your cycle and are confident a long-term fasting window won't derail your plans.

Regardless of the length of your fasting window, whether it is 12, 14, or 16 hours, the most important factor to consider is the macronutrients contained in your first meal. This meal, regardless of if it is at 7am or 12pm is technically your breakfast - the word itself means to 'break' your 'fast' - so it is vital to have a healthy, balanced meal made of wholesome, nutrient-dense foods as your first meal of any day. This doesn't mean that after your first meal that you should be binge eating on everything in sight. The eating window provides the flexibility to eat what you want when you want, but sensible choices are still recommended. A balanced first meal followed by a small snack, and a full and healthy last meal are often all that's needed to meet your calorie needs for a day. If you are a highly active person, your caloric needs will be higher, but by selecting nutrient-dense foods, you can easily meet your daily calorie requirements within an 8-hour eating window.

The 5:2 Technique

Another method of intermittent fasting is to set your schedule around five days of the week where you will eat normally, and two days where you will restrict your calories to approximately one-quarter of your daily needs—this is typically 500 calories for women and approximately 600 calories for men. You can choose the fasting days that suit you best so long as you do not do them back to back—always ensure that there is at least one non-fasting day in between your fasting days.

For the 5 days of regular eating, you don't restrict the calories or the hours for which you are eating in, but this isn't a license to overeat or indulge, you still need to practice good food choices by eating reasonable portions, nutrient-dense foods and still aiming to curb late-night snacking. On the two days of fasting, you don't have to limit the time frames that you eat in, but portion sizes are small and the total calorie intake for the day should not exceed the target you've set based on your overall needs.

If the goal is weight loss, the 5:2 Method can be helpful if the protocol is followed, by reducing the total calories consumed within the week. It will not be effective if you try and compensate on the fasting days by consuming more than what is recommended for your personal daily calorie intake.

There are no strict rules for what to eat on the fasting days - other than to be sensible and choose healthy foods. One method is to start the day with a small breakfast, then skip lunch and finish the day with a small dinner, another is to have 3 equally portioned meals at breakfast, lunch, and dinner or to skip breakfast and have the calories split between lunch and dinner. If you have tried the 16:8 Method and know you can go until 12pm on just water, this may be the best method for you as it provides the 8-12 window needed for the body to enter its fasted state and trigger the functions that can have far-reaching fasting benefits, verses simple calorie reduction. Since the calories are limited being strategic about the foods selected is vital, focus on nutrient-dense foods that are high in fiber and protein as these will help keep you feeling full for a longer period and remember, beverages count so your latte or favorite beer will be off the menu on the days you choose to be fasting.

While intermittent fasting is a safe and healthy option for most people, this method may not suit everyone due to the extended length of time in a calorie deficit and the potential psychological effects it may have on someone with a history of eating disorders. These methods are meant to be used to enhance a person's well-being— but if managing the timing and the restrictions trigger behavior that you are trying to manage around food and mental health, it is not recommended to attempt any form of fasting without consulting a mental health professional. As well, individuals who experience severe drops in blood sugar or women who are breastfeeding, pregnant, trying to conceive should all be in consultation with a doctor regarding their plans to incorporate any form of intermittent fasting into their lifestyle.

24-Hour Fast (Eat-Stop-Eat)

One method of intermittent fasting is the eat-stop-eat method, which requires you to fast completely for one 24-hour span per week. With the technique, you would fast from breakfast to breakfast, or you could go from lunch to lunch the following day. The only thing you would be able to consume in these 24 hours would be water, tea, or black coffee—although coffee would be less recommended over tea due to potential caffeine sensitivity with no other nutrients in your system. Once the 24-hour fasting window is complete, you would return to a normal eating pattern of 3 meals per day, with the occasional snack, if needed—and as always, maintaining reasonable portion sizes and nutrient-dense foods, as well as staying within the required number of calories per day.

This technique can be challenging and is danger considered an advanced technique. A 24 hour fast should not be completed unless you have already done a few weeks of the 16:8 or even the 5:2 techniques described above. It is important to understand how your body responds to fasting and to be able to recognize symptoms that may put you at risk. You may experience feelings of fatigue and headaches so if you are attempting a 24-hour fast be sure to plan your first one on a day that you are not required to do a lot of physical or mental exertion.

These effects will become less extreme with increased frequency of 24-hour fasts, and you may find you can complete one even on a more demanding day, but it is advised to plan accordingly to avoid making your fasting experience unpleasant.

If you find that this type of fasting is ideal for you - and you have no existing conditions that may be adversely affected by a 24 hour fast, such as blood sugar issues or any tendencies toward an eating disorder - you could do two 24 hour fasting periods in a week. Some people find this method the simplest way to incorporate the deeper benefits of a longer fast into their lives. While not eating for 24 hours may seem extreme, with some practice it can become second nature - take for example this schedule: Eat dinner with your family at 7pm on Monday, the next morning, have a glass of water and enjoy a cup of black coffee, then go about your day with a water bottle in hand and eat dinner again with your family at 7pm. If you have no social obligations or engagements that oblige you to eat, you could easily go an entire day without having to justify your eating - or lack of - choices and could save time and money by not requiring anything to eat. With a longer fasting window, you allow your body the opportunity to fully use up all stored energy sources and trigger the metabolic changes that produce the longer-term benefits of fasting. As always, this method may not be for everyone and should be approached with caution, track your progress, and make a note of your moods, energy levels, and any changes to your menstrual cycle. This method is not recommended for people with blood sugar issues, women who are breastfeeding, pregnant, or trying to conceive.

Warrior Method (23:1 or 20:4)

This is perhaps the most extreme intermittent fasting technique and should only be attempted if you have found some success with other methods and now want to elevate your practice or see if you can achieve more profound results. In the warrior method, you are required to fast for 20 hours of the day, leaving only a 4-hour window to consume your full caloric intake, often in one large meal at the end of the day.

This method was developed by a soldier-turned-health-and-fitness-author, who discovered that an eating plan based on survival allowed them to be focused, energetic, and able to perform under stress and at a high level of intensity, despite going against everything we have traditionally been taught about nutrition. Leaning on evolutionary data and modeling this technique after ancestors who would hunt, gather, and fight by day with only the time and resources to fuel themselves at night, this technique attempts to exemplify the life of a warrior. There have been little scientific studies done on the long-term effects of this particular technique, and the results have been anecdotal—but if you have observed favorable results with other long-term fasting plans, you might be one of the people who can find a sustainable lifestyle under the warrior diet method.

With this method—according to its creator, Ori Hofmekler—there is no need to count calories, and there are no rules as to what you should and should not eat. A warrior didn't always have a choice and often had to eat what was available. Thankfully, in this modern-day, you do have a plethora of food choices, and it is always advised to reach for nutrient-dense foods over pizza delivery. It is recommended to base your daily meal around healthy fats and a large portion of protein and to add in whole sprouted grains and veggies, finishing off the meal with fruit as a 'dessert.' Timing in the warrior diet is crucial and should be adhered to for optimal results. You may consume calorie-free beverages like water, tea, and black coffee throughout the fasting window—and if necessary, you can consume a very small amount of calories from raw vegetables and, if needed, high-fat dairy like a good quality cheese of Greek yogurt. However, these should only be used if absolutely necessary.

The benefits of the warrior diet are no different than those of the other time-restricted methods such as 16:8 or even the 5:2 Method, but it is believed that by having an extended fast these benefits may be heightened. Weight loss would be nearly certain due to the restricted calories; however, if it leads to binge eating or becomes unsustainable over time, the potential for weight gain to come back is high. Blood sugar levels will be affected and could be balanced to help control insulin sensitivity however if the extend fast causes too drastic of a drop in blood sugar it could be dangerous and the spike if insulin after consuming all calories in a short time could be disagreeable with your system. Having a solid understanding of how your body behaves in extended fasting states is a vital tool to have prior to attempting this technique.

There are also several potential downfalls that you must consider before testing this method for yourself, as this level of fasting is not appropriate for large groups of people. If you have a tendency for eating disorders, this method is not recommended, as it can lead to obsessive behavior—and if you have blood sugar issues or are a woman who is breastfeeding, pregnant, or trying to conceive, this method will put your body under immense stress and is not advised. Even if you are perfectly healthy, this method can be a challenge to follow in the modern world. With social engagements and constant access to food, it will take a great deal of self-control to maintain 20 hours of fasting every day for a long period of time. However, it isn't impossible—and those people who are capable of thriving in this lifestyle report healthy energy, strong mental clarity, and a certain freedom from the never-ending question of what to make to eat now.

CHAPTER

7

Common Mistakes to Avoid When Fasting

M any people who are just starting their fasting cycle, tend to make beginners mistake, which can result in goals not being achieved and many other hosts of things. In this chapter, we will go over the main mistakes most beginners make when they first start fasting. If you are beginning with intermittent fasting, chances are you will make those mistakes. Meaning, for it to not happen, it is best that we talk about it and show you ways to combat it. With that being said, let's talk about the first mistake.

7.1

Start intermittent fasting quickly

Many beginners make the mistake of starting intermittent fasting way too fast, and when they begin to quickly, it becomes unsustainable for them to continue with intermittent fasting. If you have started anything immediately, you might have noticed that it became tough for you to follow, which led to you not continuing. Same goes for intermittent fasting, and you need to make sure you take the right steps before you jump into following intermittent fasting. With that being said, let's talk about many ways beginner intermittent fasters tend to start too quickly. The first mistake they make is by picking a fasting protocol, which is way out of their Realm.

As we talked about before, you need to ease into intermittent fasting, especially if you're women. You cannot expect to fast for 24 hours when you have never even fasted in your life, so start small. It is always recommended that women begin with 12-hour fast, or if that sounds too intense for you can start to by meal skipping. You have to make sure that, whatever you follow it is done gradually, so you don't quit. Another way people tend to start intermittent fasting too quickly is by not Consulting the doctor. Believe it or not, their chances that you might not be healthy enough to follow intermittent fasting.

That is why it is advised that you consult a doctor before starting fasting; for example, if you have diabetes, you are not advised to begin intermittent fasting. There are many health complications which not allow you to follow intermittent fasting, that is why we always recommend you ask a doctor before you start intermittent fasting or it can be very devastating.

Beginners also tend to extend the fasting window very quickly; if you haven't fasted for more than four weeks comfortably, then it is not recommended to extend the fasting window. We need to take into consideration that for beginners, going from 12 hours to 16 hours can be a drastic difference. That is why it is always advised that you stick with a fasting protocol for an extended period, ideally for four weeks. If you make the jump of increasing hours too soon, you will notice it becomes tough for you to continue with fasting and you might give up.

7.2

Choose the wrong plan for your lifestyle

Most people, when they first start intermittent fasting, tend to pick the crazy strategy for their lifestyle. It is important that you choose the right method for your lifestyle and your goals. Intermittent fasting can be very fitting for most lifestyle. However, some plans are just better suited for some. Which is what we are going to be talking about in this section of the book, picking the right plan for your lifestyle. To simplify this process, we will make up two people and make up a fake lifestyle.

Once we have managed to do that, we will figure out which fasting protocol works best for them. The first example would be Jamie, and she is the CEO of a company. Her daily routine is, she wakes up at 5 am and heads on out to her office. She works for 10 hours a day, in and out of meetings and has barely enough time to go to the bathroom. Her job is physically demanding, and it is also very mentally demanding.

Her goal is to lose a little weight, and she also wants more mental clarity since she has been noticing mental fog sometimes. According to Jamie's lifestyle, it is highly recommended that she follows a fasting protocol which requires less than 24 hours of fasting and is supported regularly. The reason behind her fasting less than 24 hours, is that when you fast for longer than 24 hours, you tend to notice diminishing results in energy. Which is not something we want for Jamie since she has to run a company. On the other hand, she wants less mental fog and more focus.

As you know, fasting for 12 to 20 hours has shown to increase mental focus, which would make a protocol 16/8 or the 12 hours fast more feasible for Jamie. She also wanted to lose weight, which can be done following the 16 hours quickly. In future, if Jamie wants to lose more weight without losing mental focus, then she can do that by following the warrior diet instead merely because it will shorten her eating window putting here in a higher caloric deficit. To summarize, Jamie's goal was to gain more mental clarity and energy while losing some fat. Her lifestyle is very demanding.

Hence, she is required to be on her "A game" every day, which is why the 12-hour fast or the 16-hour fast will work tremendously, as it has shown to help with mental energy and losing weight. If your lifestyle sounds similar to Jamie's, then I would highly recommend you follow the 12 hours fast or the 16 hours fast. For the next case study, we will pick Amanda. She has two kids, and she works part-time. Her main goal is to lose weight as quickly as possible, but healthily, she has gained a lot of weight after her last pregnancy. Her daily lifestyle is very sedentary since her kids are not infants anymore; taking care of them is more comfortable.

She works from home part-time, and her job is straightforward going. She has had experience with fasting before, she has followed the 12 hours fast and the 16 hours fasts both for four weeks. But now she is dangerous, and she wants to lose a ton of weight quickly. Since Amanda has experience with intermittent fasting, she can go right ahead and follow the two days a week fasting protocol or the alternate day fasting protocol; these two will put her in a 20%-25% deficit for the whole week making her lose weight quickly and in a healthy manner.

To sum up, Amanda, she has a very sedentary lifestyle. Her goal is to lose the pregnancy weight quickly and to do it healthily, she has followed the 12 hours fast and the 16 hours fast before. Based on her goals and lifestyle ideally, she can start with the alternate fasting protocol or the two days a week fasting protocol. If your goals and lifestyle sound very similar to Amanda's, then you should follow the two days a week fasting protocol or the alternate day fasting protocol. Hopefully, these two examples helped you understand which fasting protocol is best suited for your lifestyle. Just remember that fasting will only help you if you can do it for a sustained period, which is why lifestyle plays a huge role in sustainability for intermittent fasting. Pick your fasting protocols accordingly.

7.3

Overeat during the eating window or too little

People make the mistake of eating a lot or too little

when following intermittent fasting, and the truth is it is straightforward to do either. People who are looking to lose weight will eat less during their eating window, thinking that it will help you lose more body fat. Whereas overeating will not make up for all the fasting, you did throughout the day. Which is why it is imperative that you do none, so in this section, we will teach you how to make sure you aren't doing either when following an intermittent fasting protocol.

The first way to not mess up on overeating would be to make sure that you are counting your macros. This is one of the best ways to make sure you stay on track with your eating habits during your fasting windows. When you have calculated your macros and following them accordingly, you will have a lot better chance of not under eating or overeating during your eating window. Another way to make sure that you are not overeating is to eat slowly, and many people tend to get extremely excited when they see food in front of them during their eating window. It is best advised that you don't indulge in them and more than you should.

Now, even though fasting allows you to eat whatever you want when you break your fast, it still essential to make sure you eat correctly. You see if you try and eat junk food and try and hit your macros, it would be tough for you not to overeat. Let me explain how that works, as there is something called a high glycemic carb which most of the junk foods. What these high glycemic carbs are responsible for is digesting very quickly in your body, which spikes the insulin very fast.

When you absorb and shuttle the foods to quickly as you would with junk food, you will get hungry very fast, which would make you overeat. Which is why it is best advised that you eat foods which have a lower glycemic index like most healthy meals tend to have. Another thing these healthy foods will help you with would be the fiber, making you feel fuller through the day. Now that we know how not to overeat, let's talk about how to make sure that you aren't under-eating. The first way to make sure that you aren't under-eating would be by counting macros, and this will help you make sure that you are hitting all your calories for the day. Counting macros will ensure you don't under-eat and you don't overeat, it goes hand in hand.

Now, this is the only way to avoid under-eating let's talk about some of the signs you might be experiencing if you under-eat when fasting. The first sign you might notice is that you feel very weak when working out if you follow a workout plan you will see that your strength has gone down which is a tail-tail sign that you are under-eating. Another way to tell that you are under-eating is if you know that you feel less energy throughout the day, rather than feeling more heat. One of the many benefits of intermittent fasting is the fact that you can get a lot more power, but it won't work if you are under-eating. So by now, you can tell that overeating and under-eating aren't optimal for fasting. Which is why you need to make sure that you stay on track with your macros when fasting, the other tips we gave you work great as well.

But do whatever works for you to ensure that you aren't under eating or overeating, and there are millions of way to go about it. Find an eating routine which helps you feel full, and allows you to eat just the right amount of calories to where you are getting closer to your goals instead of drifting away from them if your goal is weight loss or muscle gains you need to make sure your calories are the right amount. Don't make this beginners mistake as you will regret it, and now you have the tools to ensure you don't make these mistakes.

7.4
Ignore what for when

One mistake that many people following intermittent fasting make is to ignore what for when. For you to be successful with intermittent fasting, you need to make sure you don't overlook what for when. What do I mean by what for when is simple, ignoring what to do and what not to do when intermittent fasting. We will talk about things to avoid and the things not to avoid when intermittent fasting. More specifically, we will teach you how to listen to your body.

You are ignoring what for when is merely a metaphor, nonetheless an important one. First of all, when intermittent fasting doesn't jump too quickly from fasts to fasts. Most beginners make the mistake of not riding out the protocol for a substantial amount of time before they jump to conclusions. Make sure that you have done at least four weeks of following this protocol as it will show you how your body reacts to this fasting method. The next thing to make sure of would be to understand how your body reacts to certain types of fasting, as it is essential that you know so.

Before you jump the guns of upping the fasting difficultly, make sure you know how your body works. You need to remember that your body is more important than your goals, so whatever you do, you need to be aware of what your body is telling you. Don't do anything which makes you feel like you are harming your body, and as always consult with your physician before you start a fast.

7.5

Not drinking enough water

Drinking water is crucial when your intermittent fasting, is there a lot of benefits to drinking water. It also helps you care about your appetite. We will talk about the reasons why you should be drinking more water when intermittent fasting, and also show you why you might not be drinking enough water and techniques to allow you to drink more water when fasting. Many people know that water is very beneficial to humans, water help to detox your body clean out your system and also helps you curb appetite. It is crucial that you're drinking more water when fasting. Believe it or not, most of the time you're drinking a lot less water than you required to be drinking. One of the best rules of thumb to follow when you are drinking water is too drink 1 oz per pound of body weight. So if you weigh 150 lbs., you should be drinking 150 ounces of water, especially when you're intermittent fasting; as water will help you forget about food.

Many people know that when you're fasting, especially in the beginning you tend to crave a lot of food. What water will do is help you curb that appetite, so you don't break you're fast prematurely, another thing water will do detoxify your body. When your fasting you're already detoxing a lot of things, if you add more water to it, it will help you detox your body even further making it a lot healthier environment for you. Water will also increase your brain power and productivity, as you know intermittent fasting has shown to improve mental focus so once you add more water to your daily routine, you will notice more focused throughout the day.

Another thing water helps you with is that it helps you lose body weight. If you started intermittent fasting in the hopes of losing weight, then you need to drink more water. What water does, is it increase your metabolism, which equals more calories burnt throughout the day. Water will also help you clean out your complexion, so if that's what you're looking for the water will help you with that. Intermittent fasting has shown to improve with your digestive system, but once you add a sufficient amount of water to it will boost it further. Many people know that regularity in the essential thing when it comes to a healthy body, why do I help you with consistency, which will equal a better digestive system and overall well-being. Water will also help you boost your immune system, as it enables you to clean out your toxins.

When incorporated with intermittent fasting, drink more water to boost your immune system. When fasting, you might notice headaches, especially in the beginning, if you drink a sufficient amount of water throughout the day, you will not see problems. Headaches is one of the biggest concerns when fasting, many people notice problems, and to avoid that you should start drinking more water. Another matter that you might see when fasting is cramped more specifically muscle cramps. One of the ways to prevent it is to drink more water. Now I can keep going on with the benefits of drinking more water, but you get the idea to drink more water to avoid side effects from fasting that you might see.

One of the ways to ensure that you drink more water is to buy a water bottle with markings on it. First, figure out how much water you need through the day and make sure you achieve your goal of drinking a set amount of water. Another way to ensure that you drink more water is to set alarms. What many people do, set alerts on this Smartphone, and when the alarm goes off the drink a glass of water. You can do the same thing to ensure they drink enough water throughout the day, calculate the number of glasses you need to achieve your water intake goal, and then set your timer.

Choose whichever method you want to make sure that you're drinking enough water throughout the day. Not drinking enough water is one of the biggest mistakes most people make. Our body is made up of around 70% water, and to ignore that and not drink enough water and hinder your progress. Make sure you're drinking enough water, during your fast and after you break your fast. To ensure that you are optimizing your fasting endeavors and getting closer to your goals.

We have now officially completed the book. I hope you learned a lot from it as it was our goal to ensure that no stones where unturned.

We understand that fasting can be confusing and hard at first, so it is essential that you are aware of the mistakes you might or might not make. Please make sure that you have understood all the things you should so and the things you shouldn't be doing. Just be aware of the fact that there might be many things which might go wrong in the beginning, learn from your mistakes, and keep moving on forward.

Don't let small mistakes stop you from achieving your dream body, and helping you live a healthier life overall. If you need extra motivation, ask a friend to keep you on track, always let them know how important it is for you to not give up on this journey. But once again, listen to your body if you feel like fasting is harming your body then stop as your body is more important than anything else, which is why we recommend getting blood work done by a professional always before you start any plan. As always, thanks for reading this book.

8

Useful and Instant Recipes for Lose Weight

8.1 Breakfast

Walnut and Cream Bars

Servings 4
Preparation Time: 20 minutes

Ingredients

1/4 teaspoon cardamom
1 cup double cream
A pinch of grated nutmeg
A pinch of coarse salt
2 tablespoons walnut butter
2 tablespoons coconut oil
1/2 cup coarsely chopped walnuts

Directions

Put foil on a baking pan.
Combine the cardamom and double cream and put it in the baking pan.
In a separate bowl, whisk together the nutmeg, salt, walnut butter and coconut oil. Spread this over the cream mixture.
Sprinkle the walnuts on top and freeze for a quarter of an hour.
Cut into squares and enjoy!

Nutrition: 278 Calories; 2.2g Protein; 30.1g fat; 2.2g carbs; 1.1g Sugar

Creole Frittata

Servings 3
Preparation Time: 25 minutes

Ingredients

1 tablespoon olive oil
1 chopped red onion
4 ounces chopped crawfish tail meat
1 teaspoon Creole seasoning blend
1/2 cup yogurt
6 slightly beaten large eggs

Directions

Put your oven on at 3500F.
Preheat an oven-proof skillet over moderate-high heat and heat the olive oil.
Fry the onions until they are tender and then add the crawfish. Cook for 2 minutes. Sprinkle with the Creole seasoning.
Whisk the yogurt with the eggs and pour this into the skillet.
Put the skillet into the oven and cook for around 18 minutes. Cut into wedges and serve hot. Bon appétit!

Nutrition: 265 Calories; 22.9g Protein; 15.8g Fat; 7.1g Carbs; 5.2g Sugar

Party Balls with Bacon and Reblochon

Servings 5
Preparation Time: 15 minutes

Ingredients

3 ounces bacon
1/2 teaspoon paprika
1/4 teaspoon parsley flakes
6 ounces Reblochon
1 seeded and finely chopped jalapeño pepper

Directions

Cook the bacon over a medium-high flame until it has browned. Cut the bacon into small pieces.
Blend the paprika, parsley flakes, Reblochon and jalapeno pepper in your food processor. Chill this mixture in your fridge.
Once the mixture is cold, shape it into 10 balls.
Roll the balls in the chopped bacon and serve. They can be kept in the fridge for up to 3 days. Bon appétit!

Nutrition: 206 Calories; 13.4g Protein; 16.5g Fat; 0.6g Carbs; 0.3g Sugar

Panna Cotta with Mushrooms

Servings 6
Preparation Time: 15 minutes + chilling time

Ingredients

1 tablespoon butter
2 ounces chopped fresh mushrooms
1 1/3 cups heavy cream
2 teaspoons powdered unflavored gelatin
8 ounces blue cheese
1 cup sour cream
1 teaspoon Herbes de Provence
1/4 cup pecan halves

Directions

Put the butter in a pan over high heat and cook the mushrooms for 4 minutes. Stir continuously.
Add the heavy cream and gelatin and bring to the boil.
Turn the heat off and mix in the blue cheese, sour cream and Herbes de Provence. Put the mixture into 6 serving glasses and refrigerate overnight.
Decorate with pecan halves.

Nutrition: 489 Calories; 12.7g Protein; 47.4g Fat; 6.9g Carbs; 1.3g Sugar

Beef Sausage Fajita

Servings 4
Preparation Time: 25 minutes

Ingredients

1 tablespoon lard
1 teaspoon crushed garlic
2 sliced smoked beef sausage links
½ teaspoon saffron
2 sliced bell peppers
1 minced piquillo pepper
1 teaspoon fajita seasoning
2 sliced zucchinis

Directions

Preheat a wok over medium heat and warm up the lard. Cook the garlic and sausage for 8 minutes until the meat has browned.
Add the saffron, bell peppers, piquillo pepper, fajita seasoning, zucchinis and cook for 13 minutes. Stir every now and again. Serve hot.

Nutrition: 227 Calories; 7.1g Protein; 18g Fat; 7g Carbs; 4g Sugar

Fried Pizza with Cheeses and Peppers

Servings 4
Preparation Time: 15 minutes

Ingredients

2 tablespoons olive oil
1/2 cup cream cheese
1 1/4 cups shredded mozzarella cheese
1/2 cup shredded Pepper Jack cheese
2 chopped garlic cloves
2 tablespoons sour cream
10 halved cherry tomatoes
1 sliced green bell pepper
1 sliced red bell pepper
1 teaspoon oregano
Salt and black pepper, to taste

Directions

Preheat a pan over medium heat and warm the olive oil.
Add the three kinds of cheese, making sure that the bottom is covered. Cook this mixture for 5 minutes until it is golden brown and crunchy.
Put the garlic and sour cream on top of the crust and add the tomatoes and peppers. Cook for another couple of minutes.
Put a sprinkling of salt, pepper and oregano on top. Serve hot.

Nutrition: 266 Calories; 9g Protein; 23.6g Fat; 6.6g Carbs; 3.7g Sugar

Simple Cheese and Pumpkin Mousse

Servings 6
Preparation Time: 15 minutes + chilling time

Ingredients

1/2 cup erythritol
1/2 cup cream cheese
1 1/2 cups heavy cream
3 eggs
1/4 teaspoon grated nutmeg
1/2 teaspoon ground cinnamon
1/2 teaspoon ground cloves
1 1/4 cups canned pumpkin
A pinch of coarse salt

Directions

In a pan, mix together the erythritol, cream cheese and heavy cream and bring to the boil. Whisk continuously. In a bowl whisk the eggs and then add half of the cream mixture. Put this back in the pan and cook for around 4 minutes until the mixture has thickened.
Switch the heat off and mix in the nutmeg, cinnamon, cloves, pumpkin and salt. Put the mixture into 6 individual bowls and refrigerate for a couple of hours. Serve cold. Bon appétit!

Nutrition: 368 Calories; 13.8g Protein; 33.7g Fat; 5.6g Carbs; 2.1g Sugar

Quick Salami and Egg Breakfast

Servings 3
Preparation Time: 5 minutes

Ingredients

3 teaspoons melted butter
6 eggs
1 teaspoon yellow mustard
3 chopped slices Genoa salami
1/2 cup cottage cheese
1/2 cup shredded American yellow cheese
Coarse salt and ground black pepper, to taste

Directions

Take 3 mason jars and grease them with the melted butter.
Crack two eggs into each jar. Divide the yellow mustard, salami, cottage cheese, yellow cheese, salt and pepper between the jars. Put the lids on and shake the jars to make sure that everything is thoroughly combined.
Take the lids off the jars and microwave them one at a time for 2 minutes.

Nutrition: 303 Calories; 21.6g Protein; 22.4g Fat; 3.6g Carbs; 2.2 Sugar

Bacon and Turkey Meatloaf Cups

Servings 6
Preparation Time: 30 minutes

Ingredients

1 teaspoon brown mustard
1 beaten egg
2 ounces chopped cooked bacon
1 pound ground turkey
2 tablespoons chopped shallots
1 teaspoon minced garlic
Coarse salt and ground black pepper, to taste
1/2 teaspoon dried oregano
1 teaspoon dried basil
1/2 teaspoon crushed red pepper flakes
4 ounces cubed Brie cheese

Directions

Mix together the mustard, egg, bacon, ground turkey, shallots and garlic.
Sprinkle the salt, black pepper, oregano, basil and red pepper flakes onto the mixture. Combine thoroughly.
Put the mixture into muffin cups and place a cube of Brie into each cup, spreading the meat mixture over the cheese.
Put your oven on at 3500F and bake the cups for around 20 minutes. Cool for 10 minutes and then remove from the muffin cups.

Nutrition: 278 Calories; 29.2g Protein; 18.3g Fat; 1.2g Carbs; 0.2g Sugar

Strawberry Omelet the French Way

Servings 1
Preparation Time: 10 minutes

Ingredients

1/2 teaspoon ground cloves
2 tablespoons heavy cream
2 beaten eggs
1 tablespoon coconut oil
8 sliced fresh strawberries
2 tablespoons cream cheese

Directions

Crack the eggs in a mixing bowl and whisk together with cloves and heavy cream.
Preheat a pan over moderate-high heat and heat the coconut oil. Add the egg mixture and cook for around 3 minutes or until the base is cooked through.
Put the omelet on a plate and spread the cream cheese on top and toss in the strawberries. Flambé and enjoy.

Nutrition: 488 Calories; 15.3g Protein; 42g Fat; 8g Carbs; 4.4g Sugar

Turkey with Prosciutto and Mustard

Servings 6
Preparation Time: 50 minutes

Ingredients

6 4-ounce turkey fillets
3 tablespoons whole grain mustard
1 tablespoon herb-infused olive oil
2 tablespoons roughly chopped fresh parsley
1 teaspoon hot paprika
1 teaspoon tarragon
1 chopped jalapeno pepper
3 chopped garlic cloves
Salt and ground black pepper, to taste
6 slices prosciutto

Directions

Put your oven on at 3900F.
With a meat mallet, flatten the turkey fillets and rub the mustard and oil over them.
Then put the parsley on each fillet. Mix together the paprika, tarragon, jalapeno pepper, garlic cloves, salt and pepper and place some of this mixture on each turkey fillet.
Take the prosciutto and roll a slice around each fillet.
Put the fillets in a glass baking dish and cook in the oven for 35 – 45 minutes. Bon appétit!

Nutrition: 275 Calories; 44.5g Protein; 9.5g Fat; 1.3g Carbs; 0.1g Sugar

Egg Muffins with Cheese and Pancetta

Servings 9
Preparation Time: 30 minutes

Ingredients

9 slices pancetta
1/2 teaspoon dill weed
1/4 teaspoon garlic powder
1/2 cup shredded Monterey Jack cheese
A bunch of chopped scallions
9 eggs
1 tablespoon coconut oil
Sea salt and ground black pepper, to taste

Directions

Put the oven on at 3900F.
Take a 9-cup muffin pan and brush with oil. Put a slice of pancetta in each cup.
Mix together the dill weed, garlic, cheese, scallions, eggs, salt and pepper.
Put the mixture into the muffin cups and cook for 20 minutes. Bon appétit!

Nutrition: 294 Calories; 21g Protein; 21.4g Fat; 3.5g Carbs; 1.7g Sugar

Delicious Tuna Pâté

Servings 12
Preparation Time: 10 minutes + chilling time

Ingredients

1 14-ounce drained tuna in brine
½ teaspoon smoked paprika
2 ounces finely chopped cilantro
1/2 teaspoon country Dijon mustard
2 tablespoons mayonnaise
1/4 cup sour cream
1/2 cup Ricotta cheese
Coarse salt and freshly cracked mixed peppercorns, if wanted.

Directions

Mix together the tuna, paprika, cilantro, mustard, mayonnaise, sour cream, Ricotta cheese, salt and pepper. Make sure that everything is well mixed.
Grease a mold and pour in the mixture. Chill overnight.
Take the pate out of the bowl by inverting It onto a serving plate. Enjoy with slices of French toast.

Nutrition: 84 Calories; 7.9g Protein; 2.9g Fat; 1.3g Carbs; 0.2g Sugar

Porridge with Hemp Hearts and Brazil Nuts

Servings 4
Preparation Time: 20 minutes

Ingredients

2 tablespoons coconut oil, room temperature
1/4 pinch psyllium husk powder
20 drops liquid stevia
1/4 cup freshly ground flaxseed
¼ cup hemp hearts
4 lightly whisked eggs
A dash of ground cinnamon
1/4 teaspoon coarse salt
1 teaspoon pure vanilla extract
16 Brazil nuts

Directions

Put a pan on a moderate-low heat and add the coconut oil, psyllium husk powder, liquid stevia, flaxseed, hemp hearts and eggs.
Stir the mixture until it is all mixed together. Raise the heat a little and add the cinnamon, salt and vanilla extract. Cook until the porridge begins to boil.
Put the porridge into 4 bowls and top each with 4 brazil nuts. Eat while still warm.

Nutrition: 405 Calories; 14.8g Protein; 37g Fat; 6.6g Carbs; 1.5g Sugar

Waffles with Asiago and Pancetta

Servings 3
Preparation Time: 20 minutes

Ingredients

6 large-sized eggs with egg whites and egg yolks separated
1/2 teaspoon dried oregano
Kosher salt to taste
4 tablespoons ghee
1/2 teaspoon baking soda
1/2 teaspoon baking powder
3 tablespoons tomato paste
3 ounces shredded Asiago cheese
3 ounces chopped pancetta

Directions

Mix together the egg yolks, oregano, salt, ghee, baking soda and baking powder.
In another bowl, whisk the egg whites with an electric mixer until it stands in peaks. Add this to the egg yolk mixture.
Take a waffle iron, grease it and heat it up. When hot pour in some of the batter. Cook for about 3 minutes until the waffle is golden. Repeat. You should end up with 6 thin waffles.
Put one waffle back in the waffle iron and spread 1 tablespoon of tomato paste on it. Add an ounce of the cheese and an ounce of pancetta. Top with another waffle and cook until the cheese starts melting. Do this another two times and serve straight away.

Nutrition: 453 Calories; 25.6g Protein; 37g Fat; 4.5g Carbs; 2.4g Sugar

Berry Pancakes the Greek Way

Servings 4
Preparation Time: 20 minutes

Ingredients

For the Batter:
6 ounces Ricotta cheese at room temperature
1 teaspoon baking powder
A pinch of salt
5 eggs
For the Topping:
2 tablespoons coconut oil
1 cup fresh mixed berries
2 tablespoons Swerve
1/4 teaspoon freshly grated nutmeg
1/2 cup Greek yogurt

Directions

With an electric mixer, combine the Ricotta cheese with the baking powder, salt and eggs.
Put a frying pan on a moderate heat and warm up the coconut oil.
Put some of the batters in the pan and cook for 3 minutes on each side.
Once all of the pancakes have been cooked, put the fresh berries on them and add the Swerve and nutmeg. Put a big spoonful of Greek yogurt on top of each pancake.
Serve immediately!

Nutrition: 287 Calories; 14.5g Protein; 16.3g Fat; 5.5g Carbs; 3.1g Sugar

8.2 Mains

Cauliflower Soup with Seeds

Preparation Time: 10 minutes
Cooking time: 20 minutes
Serves: 4

Ingredients

2 cups cauliflower
1 tablespoon pumpkin seeds
1 tablespoon chia seeds
½ teaspoon salt
1 teaspoon butter
¼ white onion, diced
½ cup coconut cream
1 cup of water
4 oz Parmesan, grated
1 teaspoon paprika
1 tablespoon dried cilantro

Directions

Chop cauliflower and put in the saucepan.
Add salt, butter, diced onion, paprika, and dried cilantro.
Cook the cauliflower over the medium heat for 5 minutes.
Then add coconut cream and water.
Close the lid and boil soup for 15 minutes.
Then blend the soup with the help of hand blender.
Dring to boil it again.
Add grated cheese and mix up well.
Ladle the soup into the serving bowls and top every bowl
with pumpkin seeds and chia seeds.

Nutrition: calories 214, fat 16.4, fiber 3.6, carbs 8.1,
protein 12.1

Prosciutto-Wrapped Asparagus

Preparation Time: 15 minutes
Cooking time: 20 minutes
Serves: 6

Ingredients

2-pound asparagus
8 oz prosciutto, sliced
1 tablespoon butter, melted
½ teaspoon ground black pepper
4 tablespoon heavy cream
1 tablespoon lemon juice

Directions

Slice prousciutto slices into strips.
Wrap asparagus into prosciutto strips and place on the tray.
Sprinkle the vegetables with ground black pepper, heavy cream, and lemon juice. Add butter.
Preheat the oven to 365F.
Place the tray with asparagus in the oven and cook for 20 minutes.
Serve the cooked meal only hot.

Nutrition: calories 138, fat 7.9, fiber 3.2, carbs 6.9, protein 11.5

Stuffed Bell Peppers

Preparation Time: 10 minutes
Cooking time: 25 minutes
Serves: 4

Ingredients

4 bell peppers
1 ½ cup ground beef
1 zucchini, grated
1 white onion, diced
½ teaspoon ground nutmeg
1 tablespoon olive oil
1 teaspoon ground black pepper
½ teaspoon salt
3 oz Parmesan, grated

Directions

Cut the bell peppers into halves and remove seeds.
Place ground beef in the skillet.
Add grated zucchini, diced onion, ground nutmeg, olive oil, ground black pepper, and salt.
Roast the mixture for 5 minutes.
Place bell pepper halves in the tray.
Fill every pepper half with ground beef mixture and top with grated Parmesan.
Cover the tray with foil and secure the edges.
Cook the stuffed bell peppers for 20 minutes at 360F.

Nutrition: calories 241, fat 14.6, fiber 3.4, carbs 11, protein 18.6

Stuffed Eggplants with Goat Cheese

Preparation Time: 15 minutes
Cooking time: 25 minutes
Serves: 4

Ingredients

1 large eggplant, trimmed
1 tomato, crushed
1 garlic clove, diced
½ teaspoon ground black pepper
½ teaspoon smoked paprika
1 cup spinach, chopped
4 oz goat cheese, crumbled
1 teaspoon butter
2 oz Cheddar cheese, shredded

Directions

Cut the eggplants into halves and then cut every half into 2 parts.
Remove the flesh from the eggplants to get eggplant boards.
Mix up together crushed tomato, diced garlic, ground black pepper, smoked paprika, chopped spinach, crumbled goat cheese, and butter.
Fill the eggplants with this mixture.
Top every eggplant board with shredded Cheddar cheese.
Put the eggplants in the tray.
Preheat the oven to 365F.
Place the tray with eggplants in the oven and cook for 25 minutes.

Nutrition: calories 229, fat 16.1, fiber 4.6, carbs 9, protein 13.8

Korma Curry

Preparation Time: 10 minutes
Cooking time: 25 minutes
Serves: 6

Ingredients

3-pound chicken breast, skinless, boneless
1 teaspoon garam masala
1 teaspoon curry powder
1 tablespoon apple cider vinegar
½ coconut cream
1 cup organic almond milk
1 teaspoon ground coriander
¾ teaspoon ground cardamom
½ teaspoon ginger powder
¼ teaspoon cayenne pepper
¾ teaspoon ground cinnamon
1 tomato, diced
1 teaspoon avocado oil
½ cup of water

Directions

Chop the chicken breast and put it in the saucepan.
Add avocado oil and start to cook it over the medium heat.
Sprinkle the chicken with garam masala, curry powder,
apple cider vinegar, ground coriander, cardamom, ginger
powder, cayenne pepper, ground cinnamon, and diced
tomato. Mix up the ingredients carefully. Cook them for
10 minutes.
Add water, coconut cream, and almond milk. Saute the
meal for 10 minutes more.

Nutrition: calories 411, fat 19.3, fiber 0.9, carbs 6, protein
49.9

Zucchini Bars

Preparation Time: 10 minutes
Cooking time: 15 minutes
Serves: 8

Ingredients

3 zucchinis, grated
½ white onion, diced
2 teaspoons butter
3 eggs, whisked
4 tablespoons coconut flour
1 teaspoon salt
½ teaspoon ground black pepper
5 oz goat cheese, crumbled
4 oz Swiss cheese, shredded
½ cup spinach, chopped
1 teaspoon baking powder
½ teaspoon lemon juice

Directions

In the mixing bowl, mix up together grated zucchini, diced onion, eggs, coconut flour, salt, ground black pepper, crumbled cheese, chopped spinach, baking powder, and lemon juice.
Add butter and churn the mixture until homogenous.
Line the baking dish with baking paper.
Transfer the zucchini mixture in the baking dish and flatten it.
Preheat the oven to 365F and put the dish inside.
Cook it for 15 minutes. Then chill the meal well.
Cut it into bars.

Nutrition: calories 199, fat 1316, fiber 215, carbs 7.1, protein 13.1

Mushroom Soup

Preparation Time: 10 minutes
Cooking time: 25 minutes
Serves: 4

Ingredients

1 cup of water
1 cup of coconut milk
1 cup white mushrooms, chopped
½ carrot, chopped
¼ white onion, diced
1 tablespoon butter
2 oz turnip, chopped
1 teaspoon dried dill
½ teaspoon ground black pepper
¾ teaspoon smoked paprika
1 oz celery stalk, chopped

Directions

Pour water and coconut milk in the saucepan. Bring the liquid to boil.
Add chopped mushrooms, carrot, and turnip. Close the lid and boil for 10 minutes.
Meanwhile, put butter in the skillet. Add diced onion. Sprinkle it with dill, ground black pepper, and smoked paprika. Roast the onion for 3 minutes.
Add the roasted onion in the soup mixture.
Then add chopped celery stalk. Close the lid.
Cook soup for 10 minutes.
Then ladle it into the serving bowls.

Nutrition: calories 181, fat 17.3, fiber 2.5, carbs 6.9, protein 2.4

Stuffed Portobello Mushrooms

Preparation Time: 10 minutes
Cooking time: 10 minutes
Serves: 4

Ingredients

2 portobello mushrooms
1 cup spinach, chopped, steamed
2 oz artichoke hearts, drained, chopped
1 tablespoon coconut cream
1 tablespoon cream cheese
1 teaspoon minced garlic
1 tablespoon fresh cilantro, chopped
3 oz Cheddar cheese, grated
½ teaspoon ground black pepper
2 tablespoons olive oil
½ teaspoon salt

Directions

Sprinkle mushrooms with olive oil and place in the tray.
Transfer the tray in the preheated to 360F oven and broil
them for 5 minutes.
Meanwhile, blend together artichoke hearts, coconut
cream, cream cheese, minced garlic, and chopped cilantro.
Add grated cheese in the mixture and sprinkle with
ground black pepper and salt.
Fill the broiled mushrooms with the cheese mixture and
cook them for 5 minutes more. Serve the mushrooms
only hot.

Nutrition: calories 183, fat 16.3, fiber 1.9, carbs 3, protein
7.7

Lettuce Salad

Preparation Time: 10 minutes
Serves: 1

Ingredients

1 cup Romaine lettuce, roughly chopped
3 oz seitan, chopped
1 tablespoon avocado oil
1 teaspoon sunflower seeds
1 teaspoon lemon juice
1 egg, boiled, peeled
2 oz Cheddar cheese, shredded

Directions

Place lettuce in the salad bowl. Add chopped seitan and shredded cheese.
Then chop the egg roughly and add in the salad bowl too.
Mix up together lemon juice with the avocado oil.
Sprinkle the salad with the oil mixture and sunflower seeds. Don't stir the salad before serving.

Nutrition: calories 663, fat 29.5, fiber 4.7, carbs 3.8, protein 84.2

Onion Soup

Preparation Time: 10 minutes
Cooking time: 25 minutes
Serves: 6

Ingredients

2 cups white onion, diced
4 tablespoon butter
½ cup white mushrooms, chopped
3 cups of water
1 cup heavy cream
1 teaspoon salt
1 teaspoon chili flakes
1 teaspoon garlic powder

Directions

Put butter in the saucepan and melt it.
Add diced white onion, chili flakes, and garlic powder.
Mix it up and saute for 10 minutes over the medium-low heat.
Then add water, heavy cream, and chopped mushrooms.
Close the lid.
Cook the soup for 15 minutes more.
Then blend the soup until you get the creamy texture.
Ladle it in the bowls.

Nutrition: calories 155, fat 15.1, fiber 0.9, carbs 4.7, protein 1.2

Asparagus Salad

Preparation Time: 10 minutes
Cooking time: 15 minutes
Serves: 3

Ingredients

10 oz asparagus
1 tablespoon olive oil
½ teaspoon white pepper
4 oz Feta cheese, crumbled
1 cup lettuce, chopped
1 tablespoon canola oil
1 teaspoon apple cider vinegar
1 tomato, diced

Directions

Preheat the oven to 365F.
Place asparagus in the tray, sprinkle with olive oil and white pepper and transfer in the preheated oven. Cook it for 15 minutes.
Meanwhile, put crumbled Feta in the salad bowl.
Add chopped lettuce and diced tomato.
Sprinkle the ingredients with apple cider vinegar.
Chill the cooked asparagus to the room temperature and add in the salad.
Shake the salad gently before serving.

Nutrition: calories 207, fat 17.6, fiber 2.4, carbs 6.8, protein 7.8

Cauliflower Tabbouleh

Preparation Time: 10 minutes
Cooking time: 4 minutes
Serves: 4

Ingredients

1-pound cauliflower head
1 cucumber, chopped
2 tablespoons lemon juice
2 tablespoons olive oil
½ cup fresh parsley
1 garlic clove, diced
1 oz scallions, chopped
1 teaspoon mint

Directions

Trim and chop cauliflower head. Transfer it in the food processor and pulse until you get cauliflower rice.
Transfer the cauliflower rice in the glass mixing bowl. Add lemon juice and chopped scallions. Mix up the mixture.
Microwave it for 4 minutes.
Meanwhile, blend together olive oil, parsley, and diced garlic.
Mix up together cooked cauliflower rice with parsley mixture. Add mint and chopped cucumbers.
Mix it up and transfer on the serving plates.

Nutrition: calories 108, fat 7.3, fiber 3.7, carbs 10.2, protein 3.2

Stuffed Artichoke

Preparation Time: 10 minutes
Cooking time: 15 minutes
Serves: 4

Ingredients

2 artichokes
4 tablespoon Parmesan, grated
2 teaspoon almond flour
1 teaspoon minced garlic
3 tablespoons sour cream
1 teaspoon avocado oil
1 cup water, for cooking

Directions

Pour water in the saucepan and bring it to boil.
When the water is boiling, add artichokes and boil them for 5 minutes.
Drain water from artichokes and trim them.
Remove the artichoke hearts.
Preheat the oven to 365F.
Mix up together almond flour, grated Parmesan, minced garlic, sour cream, and avocado oil.
Fill the artichokes with cheese mixture and place on the baking tray.
Cook the vegetables for 10 minutes.
Then cut every artichoke into halves and transfer on the serving plates.

Nutrition: calories 162, fat 10.7, fiber 5.9, carbs 12.4, protein 8.2

Beef Salpicao

Preparation Time: 10 minutes
Cooking time: 18 minutes
Serves: 2

Ingredients

1-pound rib eye, boneless
2 garlic cloves, peeled, diced
2 tablespoons butter
1 tablespoon sour cream
½ teaspoon salt
½ teaspoon chili pepper
1 tablespoon lime juice

Directions

Cut rib eye into the strips.
Sprinkle the meat with salt, chili pepper, and lime juice.
Toss butter in the skillet. Add diced garlic and roast it for 2 minutes over the medium heat.
Then add meat strips and roast them over the high heat for 2 minutes from each side.
Add sour cream and close the lid. Cook the meal for 10 minutes more over the medium heat. Stir it from time to time.
Transfer cooked beef salpicao on the serving plates.

Nutrition: calories 641, fat 52.8, fiber 0.1, carbs 1.9, protein 42.5

8.3   Snacks

"Crocked" Button Mushrooms

Serves: 6
Preparation Time: 5 minutes
Cooking Time: 10 minutes

Ingredients

1 1/2 lbs. fresh button mushrooms, rinsed
1 cup white wine
2 Tbsp of vinegar
1/2 cup olive oil
1/2 tsp garlic powder
salt and freshly ground pepper to taste
1 dash hot pepper powder
1 pinch parsley flakes
1 pinch of dry basil

Directions

1. In a large pot, place all Ingredients and cook for 3 - 4 minutes on medium-high heat.
2. Remove from the heat and allow to cool completely.
3. Place mushrooms in colander to drain.
4. Serve or keep refrigerated.

Nutrition

Calories: 218 Carbohydrates: 4.5g Proteins: 4g Fat: 18.5g
Fiber: 1.2g

Baked Almond Crusted Zucchini Slices

Serves: 6
Preparation Time: 15 minutes
Cooking Time: 15 minutes

Ingredients

2 large zucchinis, sliced
1 cup almond flour
1 egg
Sea salt and ground black pepper to taste
1 tsp garlic powder
1 tsp onion powder
1 tsp fresh thyme (chopped fine)

Directions

1. Preheat oven to 450ºF/230ºC.
2. Line a baking sheet with parchment paper and set aside.
3. In a bowl, beat the egg.
4. In a separate bowl, combine almond flour, salt and black pepper, garlic and onion powder, thyme.
5. Dip zucchini slices in the egg and let excess drip off, drop in the almond flour mixture to coat.
6. Place coated zucchini slices onto prepared baking sheet.
7. Bake for 13 - 15 minutes flipping once.
8. Serve warm.

Nutrition

Calories: 165 Carbohydrates: 6g Proteins: 8g Fat: 13g
Fiber: 3.4g

Mini Bacon-Chicken Skewers

Serves: 6
Preparation Time: 15 minutes
Cooking Time: 35 minutes

Ingredients

2 chicken breast fillets, cut into cubes
Salt and ground pepper
10 slices of bacon
1 cup of cream cheese
1 cup of yogurt
2 Tbsp of mayonnaise
2 Tbsp of mustard

Directions

1. Cut the chicken into small pieces; season the salt and pepper.
2. In a bowl, combine mayonnaise, yogurt, mustard, and the salt and pepper.
3. Add the chicken pieces and stir.
4. Cover and refrigerate for 2 - 3 hours.
5. Preheat the oven to 360ºF/180ºC.
6. Cut bacon into bits.
7. Thread chicken and bacon on skewers one after another.
8. Place the chicken-bacon skewers in a baking dish.
9. Bake for 15 minutes, and then, turn and bake for further 10 minutes.
10. Serve hot.

Nutrition

Calories: 561 Carbohydrates: 3g Proteins: 29g Fat: 46g
Fiber: 0.2g

Grilled Goat Skewers with Yogurt Marinade

Serves: 4
Preparation Time: 20 minutes
Cooking Time: 10 minutes

Ingredients

1 lbs. boneless goat loin, cut into 1/2" cubes
Marinade
1 Tbsp lemon juice
1 cup yogurt
1/4 tsp ground ginger
1/2 tsp turmeric
1/2 tsp ground cumin
1 Tbsp ground coriander
1/2 tsp salt

Directions

1. Cut boneless goat loin, cut into 1/2" cubes.
2. In a bowl, whisk together all Ingredients for marinade. Add the goat to the bowl and stir to coat with the marinade evenly. Cover and refrigerate overnight.
3. Remove the bowl with marinated goat 15 - 20 minutes before grilling.
4. Preheat your grill to HIGH according to manufacturer Instructions.
5. Remove the meat from the marinade, and dry on kitchen paper towel. Thread goat meat on skewers.
6. Grill for about 4 - 5 minutes on each side.
7. Serve hot.

Nutrition

Calories: 131 Carbohydrates: 1.4g Proteins: 24g Fat: 3g
Fiber: 1g

Pancetta Muffins

Serves: 12
Preparation Time: 15 minutes
Cooking Time: 3 hours

Ingredients

6 slices pancetta cut in small cubes
2 cups of almond flour
2 tsp baking soda
1/4 tsp salt
2 Tbsp spring onion chopped (only white parts)
1 1/2 cup grated Parmesan cheese
1 1/2 tsp ground allspice
2 Eggs
3/4 cup almond milk (unsweetened)
1/2 cup olive oil
1 cup water for Instant Pot

Directions

1. Lightly grease a muffin cups; set aside.
2. In a bowl, stir the almond flour, baking soda, salt, allspice powder, spring onion, parmesan cheese and pancetta.
3. In a second bowl, whisk almond milk, eggs, olive oil, and salt. Combine the almond flour mixture with egg mixture and stir well.
4. Pour the batter in muffins cups (3/4 of each muffins cup)
5. Pour water to the inner stainless-steel pot in the Crock Pot, and place the trivet inside (steam rack or a steamer basket).
6. Place the muffins cups on trivet, cover and cook on HIGH for 2 - 3 hours.
7. Serve warm or cold.

Nutrition

Calories: 233 Carbohydrates: 1.5g Proteins: 8g Fat: 22g
Fiber: 0.1g

Almond Ginger Stir-Fry

Serves: 4
Preparation Time: 5 minutes
Cooking Time: 20 minutes

Ingredients

2 Tbsp olive oil
1 cup whole almonds
2 cloves garlic, halved
1 lbs. of button mushrooms
2-3 tsp minced fresh ginger
1/3 cup water
3 Tbsp coconut aminos
2 Tbsp almond flour
Salt to and d black pepper to taste

Directions

1. Heat the olive oil in large skillet over medium heat.
2. Add almonds and cook and stir for about 8 minutes until lightly browned. 3. Remove almonds with slotted spoon on a plate and set aside.
4. In a same skillet add little oil, and sauté garlic with a pinch of salt for 2 - 3 minutes.
5. Add mushrooms and ginger, and. stir-fry about 5 minutes.
6. In small bowl combine water, coconut aminos and almond flour and mix thoroughly.
7. Add the mixture to skillet; cook and toss about 2 minutes.
8. Taste and adjust the salt and pepper.
9. Serve hot.

Nutrition

Calories: 304 Carbohydrates: 8g Proteins: 17g Fat: 27g
Fiber: 5g

Chili Almond Coated Turkey Bites

Serves: 6
Preparation Time: 15 minutes

Ingredients

1 lbs. ground turkey
3 Tbsp mayonnaise
2 Tbsp onion grated
2 Tbsp parsley minced
Salt to taste
3 drops of hot pepper sauce as Tabasco (optional)
4 Tbsp ground almonds

Directions

1. In a bowl, stir all (except almonds) Ingredients until well combined.
2. Shape the mixture into small bite-size pieces and roll in ground nuts.
3. Cover and refrigerate until serving.

Nutrition
Calories: 177 Carbohydrates: 4g Proteins: 16.5g Fat: 12g
Fiber: 0.8g

Cold Cheese Dip

Serves: 6
Preparation Time: 15 minutes
Cooking Time: 5 minutes

Ingredients

4 bacon slices, cooked and crumbled
2 Tbs chopped green onions
1 cup shredded swiss or beaufort (or gruyere) cheese
3/4 cup cream cheese, softened
1/2 cup mayonnaise
1/2 tsp yellow mustard
1/8 tsp freshly ground black pepper

Directions

1. In a skillet fry the bacon until crispy; remove from heat and let cool on kitchen paper towel.
2. Chop green onion in thin slices.
3. Combine all Ingredients in a large bowl, along with crumbled bacon, and stir with a spoon.
4. Cover ball with plastic membrane and refrigerate for 2 hours.
5. Serve.

Nutrition

Calories: 355 Carbohydrates: 3g Proteins: 9.5g Fat: 33g
Fiber: 0.1g

Creamy Chicken Topped Cucumbers

Serves: 18
Preparation Time: 15 minutes

Ingredients

8 oz chicken breast, finely chopped
4 Tbsp of mayonnaise
2 Tbsp of yellow mustard
2 Tbsp green onions, finely chopped
1/8 tsp garlic powder
Ground black pepper to taste
3 cucumbers cut into thin slices

Directions

1. Line a shallow dish with the parchment paper.
2. Slice cucumbers into thin slices and place on a dish.
3. In a bowl, combine chicken, mayonnaise, mustard, green onion, garlic powder and ground black pepper.
4. Top each cucumber slice with 1 or 1 1/2 tablespoon chicken mixture.
5. Refrigerate for 2 hours or more and serve.

Nutrition

Calories: 28 Carbohydrates: 2g Proteins: 1.5g Fat: 2g
Fiber: 0.5g

Baby Bella Mushrooms Stuffed with Olives

Serves: 10
Preparation Time: 15 minutes

Ingredients

20 Baby Bella Mushrooms
2 cups cream cheese, at room temperature
20 olives green or black
1/4 cup fresh parsley finely chopped
1/2 tsp Salt and ground black pepper

Directions

1. In a bowl, stir well cream cheese.
2. Shape balls from cream cheese and put one olive in a center.
3. Place mushrooms on a serving plate and place the cream cheese balls on each mushroom.
4. Generously sprinkle with chopped parsley.
5. Refrigerate for 4 - 6 hours.
6. Serve cold.

Nutrition

Calories: 179 Carbohydrates: 3,5g Proteins: 4g Fat: 17g
Fiber: 0,7g

Curry Seasoned Almonds

Serves: 12
Preparation Time: 15 minutes
Cooking Time: 5 minutes

Ingredients

1 Tbsp curry powder
1 Tbsp chili powder
1 1/2 Tbsp celery salt
1 Tbsp stevia sweetener, granulated
2 Tbsp of olive oil
1 lbs. of whole almonds

Directions

1. In a bowl, combine curry and chili powder, celery salt and stevia; set aside.
2. Heat the olive oil in a large frying skillet and fry almonds for 2 - 3 minutes (stir frequently).
3. Sprinkle almonds curry mixture and stir until well coated.
4. Transfer almonds on a baking pan and let cool for 15 minutes.
5. Serve.

Nutrition

Calories: 222 Carbohydrates: 7g Proteins: 7.2g Fat: 20g
Fiber: 4g

Dark Avocado Bars

Serves: 8
Preparation Time: 15 minutes

Ingredients

1/2 cup coconut oil, melted
3 Tbsp of coconut butter
2 medium avocados
1/3 cup dark cacao nibs (60 - 69% cacao solid)
1/4 cup stevia sweetener, granulated
1 tsp pure vanilla extract

Directions

1. Melt coconut oil and coconut butter in microwave oven for 10 - 13 seconds.
2. Line with parchment paper a large shallow dish and pour the coconut mixture.
3. Freeze for 4 hours or overnight.
4. Remove dish from freezer and cut into pieces. Serve.
5. Store in a container and keep in freezer.

Nutrition

Calories: 214 Carbohydrates: 5.5g Proteins: 2g Fat: 22g
Fiber: 3.7g

Fried Kale Fritters

Serves: 4
Preparation Time: 10 minutes
Cooking Time: 10 minutes

Ingredients

1 cup almond flour
1/4 cup water
1 green chili chopped finely
1/4 tsp red chili powder
1/4 tsp turmeric powder
1 tsp cumin seed powder
Ground black pepper
1 tsp cooking soda
1 bunch of kale finely chopped
1/2 cups olive oil for frying

Directions

1. In a large bowl, combine the almond flour, water, chili pepper and the spices and stir well,
2. Add kale to the almond flour mixture and toss to coat well.
3. Heat the oil in a large frying pan on high-medium heat.
4. Scoop a tablespoon of the mixture and place in a pan.
5. Fry kale until golden color and crisp from both sides.
6. Remove kale fritters with slotted spoon and place on plate lined with absorbent paper.
7. Serve hot.

Nutrition

Calories: 128 Carbohydrates: 9g Proteins: 4g Fat: 15g
Fiber: 2.6g

Frozen Coconut Mocha Smoothie

Serves: 2
Preparation Time: 10 minutes

Ingredients

2 cups unsweetened coconut milk canned
2 tsp instant coffee granules
1 tsp cocoa powder
2 - 3 Tbsp of natural sweetener such Stevia, Truvia etc.
1/2 tsp vanilla extract
1 cup Ice cubes crushed (optional)

Directions

1. Add all Ingredients in a blender and blend until combined well.
2. Pour the mixture in a freezer-safe container and freeze for about 4 hours.
3. Remove from the fridge 15 minutes before serving.
4. Give a good stir and serve.

Nutrition

Calories: 456 Carbohydrates: 8g Proteins: 5g Fat: 48.5g
Fiber: 1g

Goat Cheese Spread

Serves: 6
Preparation Time: 10 minutes

Ingredients

1 cup goat cheese crumbled
1 cup of cream cheese
1/4 cup plain yogurt
1 clove of garlic sliced
1 Tbsp chopped chives
1/2 tsp dried thyme
Salt and freshly ground black pepper to taste

Directions

1. In a bowl, combine all Ingredients until thoroughly combined.
2. Refrigerate the mixture for 3 - 4 hours.
3. Serve cold.

Nutrition

Calories: 143 Carbohydrates: 3.5g Proteins: 13g Fat: 8.5g
Fiber: 3g

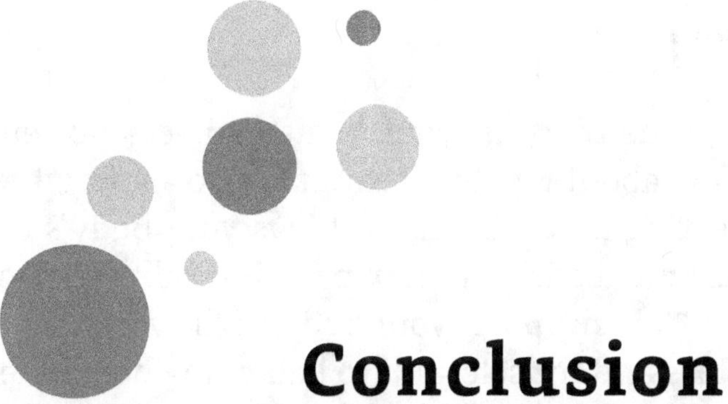

Conclusion

The truth is: your healthy diet is not entirely about what you eat. It is also about when you eat! By eating in a way that follows your body's natural rhythms and needs, you maximize its ability to function healthily. This supports your body with everything from weight loss and muscle gain to balancing hormones and blood sugar levels. There are many different benefits that you stand to gain when you monitor not only what you eat, but when.

Perhaps one of the best parts of intermittent fasting is that this unique diet does not require you to give up on anything that you truly enjoy eating. Instead, you simply change when you eat and enjoy less healthy food choices in moderation. Of course, if you prefer to combine intermittent fasting with another diet, such as the ketogenic diet, then you will have adjusted food requirements. However, the intermittent fasting diet itself does not require you to adjust your food intake to meet any specific needs.

After you have read this book, it is important that you go read my "Keto Meal Prep" book! If you are going to go ahead and adopt the keto diet as well, this book is going to massively support you in doing so. That way, you can understand the benefits of intermittent fasting and the keto diet together, as well as how you can embrace both of them to maximize your health benefits.

You do not want to find yourself taking on a new diet only to have frustrating and challenging symptoms such as headaches, fatigue, and stomach aches. This will make the transition painful and, likely, unsustainable as well. Shocking your body in this way is not healthy or helpful. Instead, take it easy and move at a pace that you can reasonably handle. Remember, this is a complete lifestyle change so you can take your time. As long as you are consistently moving forward towards your goal, consider it a success.

It is also important that you take the time to regularly monitor your symptoms and pay attention to your needs. Listen to your body and what it is telling you, as this will support you in really embracing the diet in the most powerful way possible. You do not want to find yourself struggling to succeed because you have made it too challenging for yourself. Going slower and learning to truly listen to your needs now will make your long-term goals far more achievable and sustainable.

Lastly, if you enjoyed this book and felt that it supported you in making the transition to intermittent fasting as a woman, I would like to ask that you please take a moment to leave an honest review on Amazon Kindle. Your feedback would be greatly appreciated.

Thank you, and best of luck with your intermittent fasting!

www.ingramcontent.com/pod-product-compliance
Lightning Source LLC
Chambersburg PA
CBHW070705250726
48662CB00001B/261